ELDERGIVERS

gratefully acknowledges the originating, encouraging and sustaining influence of the clergy and members of The Episcopal Church of St. Mary the Virgin in San Francisco on the growth and development of the organization. The Reverend Richard Fowler and a handful of parishioners started visiting residents at Golden Gate Healthcare Center in 1985 and Fr. Fowler's successor, The Reverend Jason Parkin, and a faithful band of volunteers led by The Reverend Dr. Everett Powell and Beverly Barrows continue to do so today.

A recent generous donation by St. Mary's has helped underwrite the printing of this second volume.

nine lives

uncovering the wealth of life stories within our nursing homes

Volume Two of the Life Stories Program

Kathleen Barrows, Editor and Project Coordinator
Brent Nettle, Executive Director, ELDERGIVERS

Contributors: Margaret S.A. Bacon, Kathleen Barrows, Michele Bigley, Victoria S. Cormack, Rebekah Eppley, Lisa Ko, Trena Noval, Ned Schaub and Cleavon Smith

Photography - Guy Poole
Book Design - John Kuzich

ELDERGIVERS
Connecting the Generations

Printed in the United States of America
First Edition

ISBN 0-9742262-1-1

Contents

Editor's Notes

Even when her one-hundred-year-old memory began to fade, to Julia I was always "the person who tells people's stories." Julia was the elder I interviewed for *Nine Lives Volume 1*. A copy of the book rested beside the urn of her ashes at the celebration of her life. I needed no more than that to convince me that I could take on the task of coordinating this second volume of *Nine Lives*.

Following in the footsteps of Sarah Merrill—who developed the idea for this series with the Executive Director of ELDERGIVERS, Brent Nettle—was an unsettling thought, but I realized I had some ideas on how to expand on the first volume. I knew firsthand my own frustrations in trying to document Julia's life. Relying too much on just getting the facts right, I had failed to capture the effect of the friendship that had magically formed between us. With Volume 2, I hoped to impart a new vision to better convey to others what can happen when "strangers" connect across age barriers.

For this second volume, Brent and I also knew we wanted a group of elders and writers representing diverse backgrounds—different ages, life experiences, writing interests, and ethnicities. Our "elders" vary in age from sixty-two to ninety-nine; our writers from twenty-nine to fifty-six. The elders live in long-term care facilities that range from Laguna Honda—San Francisco's original alms house—to The Heritage, a stately and elegant architectural landmark in the same city's affluent Marina district.

These stories include accounts of living the farm life in the South in the early 1900s; growing up Japanese-American in California; nurturing nuclear and extended families; surviving in the U.S. as an immigrant; facing discrimination for the color of one's skin; interviewing famous people the likes of David Ben Gurion; and researching the lives of sixteenth century historical figures.

For the most part, the stories represent what was recounted to the writer. We wanted to capture the elders' lives as they themselves remembered them. In a few cases, however—at the request of families or to clarify doubts—friends, relatives and published materials were consulted to supplement the narrative.

The accounts are told by writers who also have their own stories—of sorting out their ethnic identity, of learning the value of slowing down in a speeded-up world, of finding the parents and grandparents they never had, and of discovering some of themselves in their elders. They are poets, journalists, budding novelists, and creative non-fiction writers. We wanted diverse tales told in diverse styles and we got them.

Faced with unexpected challenges, it took over a year and a half to put together this book. There were the unavoidable risks of working with frail elders, all of whom were identified by Brent through his network of people who work on a day-to-day basis in Bay Area nursing homes. One elder was diagnosed with early-stage Alzheimer's shortly after being linked with her writer. Another fell ill and had to drop out of the project. Still another was moved from one facility to another in the middle of the project. A quote of Theodore Roethke eventually became my motto: "What we need is more people who specialize in the impossible."

The team of volunteer writers really did learn to "specialize in the impossible." For three writers it took an hour just to get to the long-term care facilities of their elders, and one even sacrificed her Saturday mornings for the long trek. Others squeezed in their visits after long eight-to-ten hour workdays. And that was just the visiting—there were the tape transcriptions, the note taking, the journal entries, and the painstaking process of writing.

For me, the process was as important as the actual end product. My personal measure of the success of the project was how many of the writers would continue to visit their elders, even after the "data collection" had ended. Over half of the group continues to do so, now viewing the elders as friends and mentors.

The writers worked with no model. We asked only that they maintain a journal of the process, and, if possible, tape the interviews. There really is no model for doing this kind of work, which spans the fields of gerontology, oral history, social work, ethnography, and creative writing. Throughout the project, we simply recommended books to the writers that might inspire them or help in the process. (We've included them as an appendix.)

How do you approach strangers, who have lived two or three times longer than you, to ask them to share the stories of their lives? The books on anthropology and oral history don't tell you how to delve through the folds of a brain with millions of memories tucked inside. Nor do they prepare you for the smell of illness and old age in the nursing homes, for the tears that inevitably fall, or for that far-away look in the eyes clouded by cataracts. Nothing seems to offer clues on how to un-jumble the mass of recollections into an interesting and coherent whole. And so we asked only that the pieces come from the heart.

There will always be some moments from this project that stand out—like the image of ninety-nine-year-old Mildred, sitting up in the bed she has occupied for years. With the two teeth that still remain in her mouth, she's eating a piece of pecan pie chatting with her writer, Cleavon Smith. He's pleased that the birthday pie he baked her that morning has passed her approval.

And then there were the unexpected almost miraculous coincidences—what Helen, the elder I interviewed, would call "co-innocences." When I met Lorna De Sosa, whose story begins this volume, I mentioned Helen's name. She burst into tears: Helen and Lorna had been good friends and neighbors. Neither knew that the other was still alive, but they lived in nursing homes ten minutes apart by car. Though Helen has since died, the stories of the longtime friends come together in this *Nine Lives* volume.

And there have been lessons learned. I now understand that when confined to a wheelchair, a ten-minute ride can be like traversing a continent. Because of transportation problems or distance, it can be an equally daunting challenge for the relatively healthy spouses of elders in nursing homes to visit their loved ones.

At the same time, in a seeming contradiction, the world of elders in nursing homes doesn't have to be as isolated as it might seem to us, the outsiders. The world in which our elders grew up was much smaller and slower than ours today. But by projects like this, we can help make the world of these elders, and our own, smaller again.

After all, that's what this project is about—the connections. When I told Helen that her friend Lorna would be part of this volume also, she said it was a "miraculous happening." She then went on to say: "You know my definition of a miracle? It's two people who want something and it's impossible, and they get it at the last minute." I like to think that the unexpected friendships between writers and elders that this project can set up are another one of those miracles.

Kathleen Barrows
Editor and Project Coordinator
Nine Lives, Volume 2

Introduction

Even in the face of an obvious obsession with all things young and new, one could conclude that we Americans also have a fondness and respect for what is old.

I read, for example, of environmentalists who are passionate about preserving original-growth forests. These individuals are known to chain themselves to soaring conifers that have existed for hundreds and even thousands of years to save them from the rip-saw "greed of corporate interests." I applaud their efforts. Our cathedral forests provide a soul balm that nothing else can.

While my own decorating inclinations (such as they are) lean more towards the modern, I am aware of considerable numbers of people who prefer living spaces that reflect earlier periods. In San Francisco, for instance, architectural preservationists wage an energetic battle to maintain private and public Victorian-era buildings. The human scale and muted colors of a nineteenth century brick or shingle structure or the warm glow of a polished centuries-old table or chair can offer a sense of intimacy and calm stability in the midst of what is otherwise cool, impersonal and transient.

As a former Detroiter, I find it difficult to walk by a display of automobiles from the 1920s, 30s and 40s just a block from my office without stopping to admire the obvious patience and meticulous care involved in their restoration.

Yes, there is a very certain proclivity among Americans to think of age in positive terms—as long as the object of our attention is *inanimate*. We seem to relate easily to an ancient tree or forest, an old building, a piece of antique furniture or a vintage car.

Our motivations are less clear when the object of our attention is *animate*—a human being. Unlike other more traditional cultures, North Americans continue to marginalize adults as they grow older.

In the two plus years since Volume 1 of *Nine Lives* was printed, I have seen small but definite signs of a growing openness and optimism about aging in this country. Closer notice is being paid to older people.

The increasing numbers of feature articles about the elderly in local and national media illustrate my point. These articles chronicle not only the outwardly active and useful lives that elders continue to lead in the community, but also explore and disclose the interior terrain of their lives—the hard-won moral, emotional and intellectual lessons that can arise out of longer lives and deeper experience.

Recent generations have neglected these life-lessons of our elders for too long and the resulting spiritual impoverishment of our society is all too evident. The prospect of tapping into and sharing the rich resources of age so as to nurture and nourish the wider community is exciting.

But there are still corners of our culture where the elderly remain largely ignored—corners in which the simplest and yet most profound lessons of the human condition wait to be discovered. Like those patient and persistent lovers of music and literature who every now and then turn up some long-overlooked Mozart composition or Shakespeare manuscript, there is treasure to be found in the unlikeliest of places by those who have an affection for the elderly and a passion for restoring their value to society.

It is to our shame that more than 60% of nursing home residents in the United States never have a visitor. And there is anecdotal evidence, at least in the San Francisco Bay Area, that this sad percentage is going up, not down. There seem to be fewer visitors in nursing homes today than in the past.

I wonder if this trend might not be related to another development. Since 2003, when Volume 1 of *Nine Lives* was published, nursing home populations have generally become frailer, both mentally and physically. For many people, the thought of visiting such elders and facing the declining health that advanced age may bring becomes even less appealing.

Both developments should raise serious questions.

What if, for instance, there were more visitors in nursing homes—more individuals who love animate old objects? What if these individuals have eyes that are capable of seeing beyond the declining physical abilities of elders so as to look into their hearts; visitors who have ears that hear beyond the complaints of old brains and bodies and truly listen to the stories these elders yearn to share with someone else? Could this greater interest in nursing home residents help to arrest their premature slide into frailty?

It is probably no coincidence that the elders who agreed to participate in this second volume are those who, for the most part, continue to maintain connections with the community. Most had vital relationships before entering a nursing home and have remained willing—even eager—to make new friends.

One of the intents of the *Nine Lives* series is to encourage those of us who value what is old to take the necessary practical steps to preserve what is best about animate old age. We have tried to seek out those at the farthest reaches of the human condition to bring them back to the center and help harvest their hard-earned lessons for the benefit of the whole human family.

The generous and caring writers and elders who made Volumes 1 and 2 possible provide a model for the rest of us. Their friendships promise a more meaningful old age for everyone and a truly inclusive society, especially blessed by the gifts of its oldest members.

Brent H. Nettle
Executive Director
ELDERGIVERS
San Francisco, California

nine lives

uncovering the wealth of life stories within our nursing homes

LORNA DE SOSA

Salem Lutheran Home
Oakland, California
with
Trena Noval

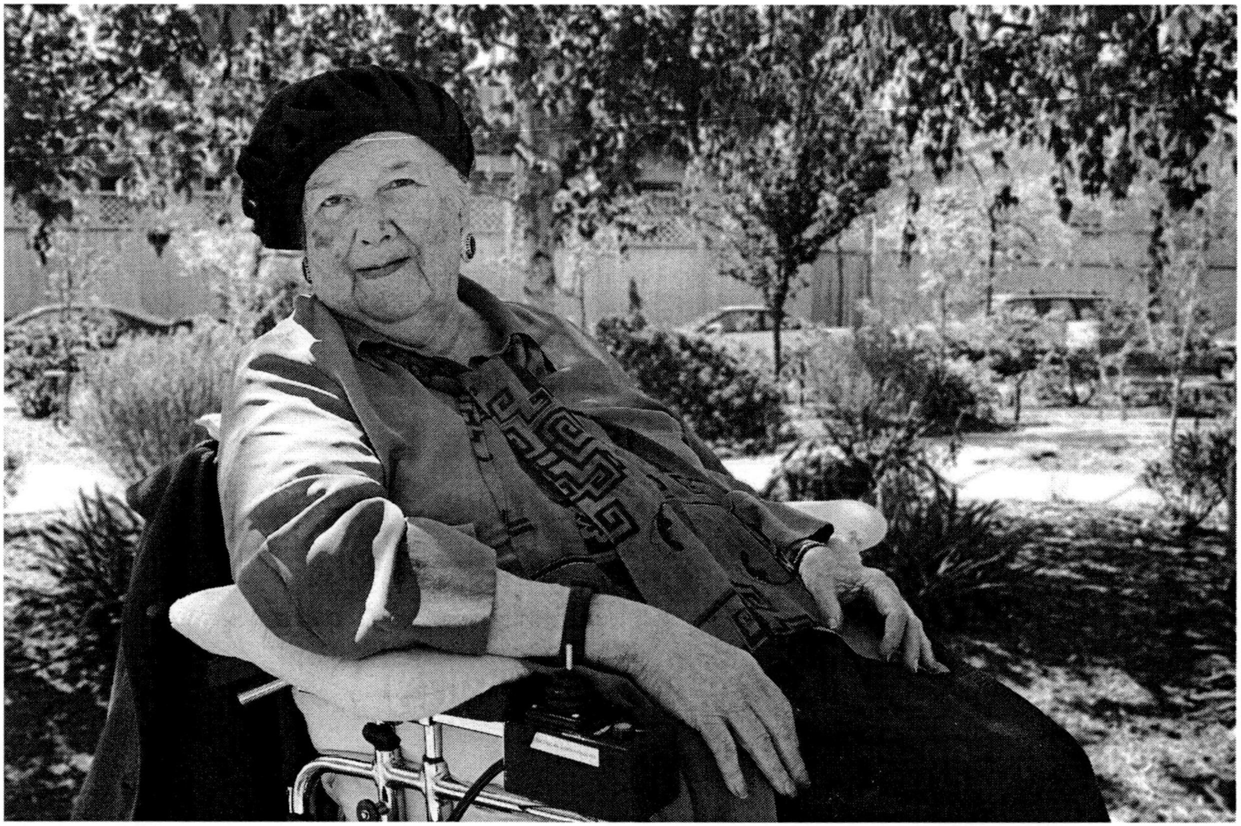

"For me, life is never ordinary"

It is early October and one of those balmy Indian summer fall days in the Bay Area. I am driving back from a long weekend away, my windows down, the wind whipping through my hair and I am giddy, tickled with my unusually clear mind and well-rested body. My cell phone beeps me a message. It's from Lorna. "Hello Trena? Are you there? Oh, that's right. You must be in Arizona. Is it Arizona? Well, I hope you are having a good time—well, not a good time but an interesting time. And I hope the moon is big and full and beautiful for you. See you when you get back." An Ansel Adams image of a big full moon over New Mexico floods my head and I know Lorna has had the same vision when she left her message—the sweeping spans of the desert landscape on a clear night.

Lorna De Sosa is charming, witty and as complex a woman as I have ever met. She doesn't miss a beat.

Lorna and I began our friendship in a twenty-first century way—through a series of messages and conversations on our cell phones. On visits, I'd follow her around the grounds of the Salem Lutheran Home in Oakland, trying to keep up with her as she zipped down hallways and outside along garden paths, driving her wheelchair that seemed turbocharged. She tells me she likes the feeling of speed. At age ninety-one, she has embraced the modern world. She is "plugged in." She carries her cell phone with her at all times—her way of navigating the world outside that she misses so desperately. On occasion I will call her and her aide, Martha, will answer her cell phone and put me on hold while she finishes a conversation on the land-based line in her room. Lorna welcomes the global communication she can have with modern technologies at the facility. She sits frequently at the computer in the library, researching topics of interest, tracking down old friends and checking her e-mail.

Lorna De Sosa is charming, witty and as complex a woman as I have ever met. She doesn't miss a beat. The first day I meet her, she makes it clear that she is a busy woman and has "business" that she conducts by phone on most days of the week. I wondered what kind of business. She is mysterious about her dealings in the world and by the end of our first meeting, it seems like she wants to keep it that way for as long as she can.

The first morning we meet, she is in her room, sitting on her bed in her bathrobe, eating fruit from a yellow bowl. She's surrounded by posterboards full of photographs with hand-written descriptions of different moments in her life—in Cuba, in Paris, with her family and friends, and as a glamorous young actress. But there is one photo in particular that stands out. It is of Lorna in a big floppy straw hat, feet bare, standing on the beach at Santa Cruz. She once tells me that she loves the sea, that she is an "ocean woman." In this picture, the water laps up, creating small fans that are hugging her ankles. She looks elated to be in this place and holds up in the air a long leggy piece of seaweed, with her arms stretched high. Playful and engaged in the moment, she looks straight into the camera with confidence and trust as though it were a dear friend that she was sharing an extraordinary day with, a big grin of sheer joy on her face. These displays, homemade, hang in her room for Lorna to celebrate her life.

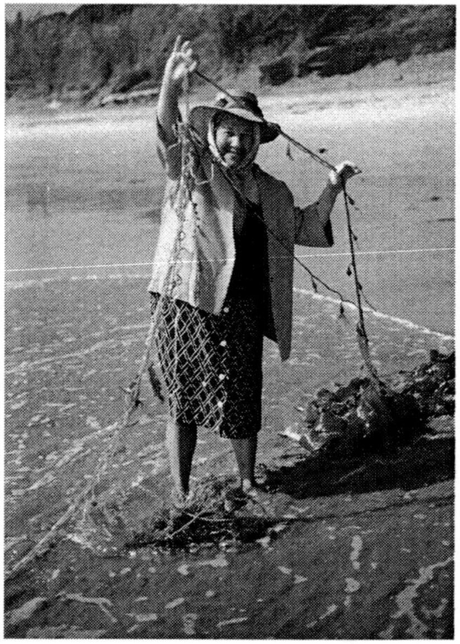

Lorna at the beach

She looks up from her bowl of fruit and greets me with a cheerful hello that bares a tinge of embarrassment in her eyes, suddenly aware that she has forgotten our meeting date. It seems as though she has been caught a little off-guard, and immediately apologizes, for both her memory slip and her informal appearance. Then without a lapse or a pause, Lorna launches into outlining her busy life, indicating the days of the week that she will be tied up making phone calls or has appointments with visitors. We get down to business right away and hammer out a visiting schedule on our calendars, plugging each other's phone numbers into our cell phones. Lorna insists that the next time I see her she will be properly dressed and wearing one of her large flamboyant hats. We giggle together about the unexpected visit like two old friends.

True to form, when we meet the following week, she is wearing a beautiful silk shirt—gold, light brown and purple paisley—secured with a garnet brooch. Her long black skirt ends in a Spanish ruffle, and she wears a flamboyant deep-purple knit hat, adorned with a large pink rose. Purple stone earrings dress her ears to complete the color scheme, and her lips are lined with a deep red lipstick—Lorna wouldn't start a day without her lipstick. From that day forward, each time we meet she is dressed as if she were greeting royalty. This care in her appearance, I soon come to find out, is a daily ritual. She has a deep sense of pride and, true to her theatrical roots as an actress and public figure, a deep commitment to fashion as well.

After a few visits, I realize that Lorna is not a morning person—she needs her mornings to collect her thoughts and wake up to the world. So we agree to meet in the late afternoons. Sometimes we talk on the phone in the late evenings. These are Lorna's preferred hours. She is a night owl—wise and looking over her domain, keeping on top of the world through her large web of phone and e-mail connections, watching the nightly news, listening to the night sounds and observing, always observing.

In one of our early meetings, we sit outside in one of the many beautiful gardens at Salem Lutheran Home. In this particular spot, there is a heavy wooden Mexican table and chair set, carved with big blossoming roses. Lorna lived a large part of her life in Cuba and loves sitting at this table. It reminds her of some of the gardens she spent time in while living in Havana. As we exit the building, Lorna points her wheelchair in the direction of the table and chairs, inhales deeply and whispers "Hello, world." It's a mantra I would hear her say during many visits, as we would stroll out of the building into the gardens at the facility. Settling in, I look at her and she seems to fit right into the mood of the furniture. She looks around and notes the change in the trees. "Every day they look different; they change like each one of them has a specific personality and daily mood," she reflects. The gardens are like a diary for her, noting time and the passing of seasons. These are her places of sanctuary, for reflection and meditation, to think, remember and imagine as she writes the stories of her life in her head. It is how she stays connected to the world at large and to nature, which she sees as an extension of herself.

The gardens are like a diary for her, noting time and the passing of seasons. These are her places of sanctuary, for reflection and meditation, to think, remember and imagine.

The sun is out and the air is starting to turn that cool autumn crisp. We are bundled in sweaters and she begins to tell me about her life. "I am a true Buckeye," Lorna announces. Born in Cincinnati, Ohio, in 1913, she was the only child of a successful businessman and a well-admired actress, writer and philanthropist. Lorna talks of her parents with great admiration and love, and describes her childhood as a good one—a simple one, filled with adventure and creativity. Her parents' love was one of great passion and friendship until the untimely death of Lorna's mother at the age of forty-three. At the time of her mother's unexpected illness, pneumonia following a gall bladder operation, Lorna was just starting college and returned home to be at her bedside. She was devastated to find her in the hospital in a protective tent that made it impossible to even touch her hand. Her mother died there in the presence of Lorna and her father. "Everyone loved her

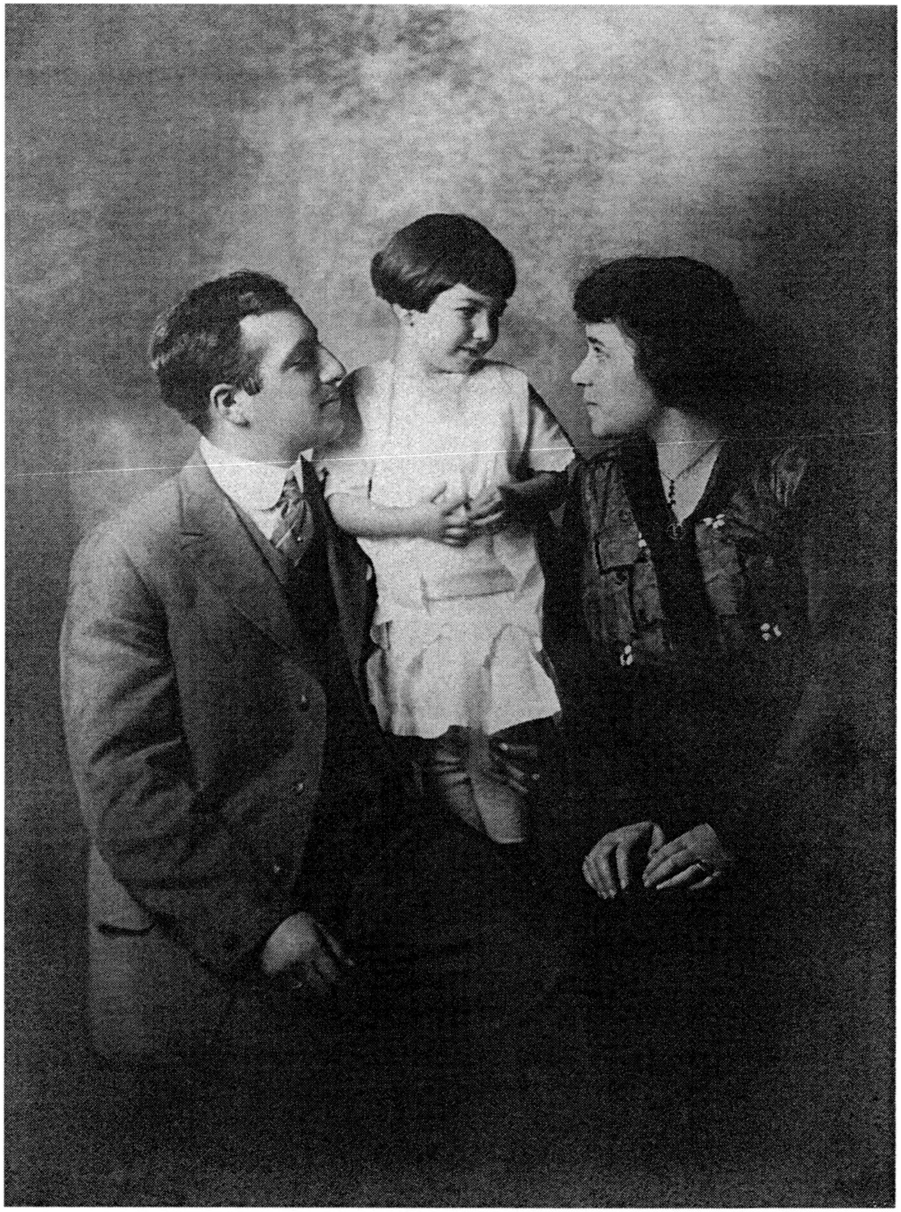

Lorna with her parents

[my mother] no matter where she was. She was magic and charming and vivacious. I remember she would always make you laugh, not with jokes but just with her good wit, and she was beautiful. I was the only child, so I was a little princess, and they didn't spoil me in that sense. I mean a little princess in their hearts. When she died, at her funeral—you'd think that she was some kind of a politician. There were just blocks and blocks of people." Lorna's memories of her mother are still very alive in her mind and as she talks, tears fill her eyes. It is clear that she still holds a deep sadness about losing such a beloved figure at a young age, but she struggles against the emotion that so often overcomes her. "Hey, Lorna," she chides herself. "Now you just stop that, Lorna—just behave."

"Everyone loved her [my mother] no matter where she was. She was magic and charming and vivacious."

Nearly four years ago my father died of cancer. He was my confidante, advisor, my hero and my biggest fan. He, like Lorna's mother, still had a lot of life to live. His loss was a difficult one for me and I have never really been able to reconcile his death in my heart. I always thought that in time it would be okay, that it would be easier to think about him and tell stories about his life to my son without feeling that my body was welling up with sadness. As I watch Lorna's reaction to her mother's death this afternoon, I can't help but wonder if after all these years, the sorrows I feel may never dispel—that they might stay deeply carved in my heart the way Lorna's mother's memory and loss has been permanently carved in hers. Lorna catches her breath again and continues her story.

Lorna tells me that her mother was one of the greatest influences on her life, the one who really helped to nurture her professional life in theater and writing: "She was an artist, but in the Victorian era. It was difficult for women to be taken seriously then in creative careers. She was as talented as the well-known actress from that time, Minnie Maddern Fiske." Fiske, a famous, red-haired actress, well-known for her portrayals of Henrik Ibsen's heroines, saw Lorna's mother perform in a local high school play while she was traveling through Ohio with a stock theater company. "She saw enormous talent in my mother's performance and asked her to come and work with her in her stock company," explains Lorna, "but my grandfather was against this."

And so Lorna's mother, the dutiful daughter that she was, conceded to her father's wishes. But she made up for the lost opportunity and her longing for the theater with her writing. "My mother wrote tremendously witty things and did all kinds of artistic things. And [I remember] also her love of sharing—for people, philanthropic things—giving of herself and doing all kinds of things for people, and the way she lived, leading a social life that was very creative." Lorna's voice trails off, as she holds on to that memory. It's as if it were a moment unfolding in slow motion in her head—watching her mother move through a group of people at a party, throwing her head back with laughter and seeing her magnetic smile again. After her mother's death, Lorna recalls, people would smile immediately and tell wonderful stories whenever her mother's name came up in conversation.

Lorna's father was a manufacturer. He owned and managed one of the largest bronze factories in Ohio. "As a child, his factory was thrilling to me," Lorna recalls. "Maybe that is where some of my theatrical background comes from, not only my mother, but all those visits to my father's factory. It was the most exciting thing. The whole floor of the factory was a big foundry and you would see them pouring copper and there were all of these flames. It was so exciting and then there would be a number of artists and designers molding it. It was called Newman Manufacturing Company." The factory produced many ornate and decorative copper and bronze light posts, large decorative gates and doorways, ornaments and replicas of historical figures for hotels, ships, theaters and buildings for sale in cities across the country. Lorna's father recounted to her what happened when he traveled to Louisiana to install large copper doors for the state capitol building. "At the time of the installation, archeologists were working in the same area of Baton Rouge and they unearthed two coffins that were from the early Spanish colonization of the area. And inside these coffins were a man and women—a bride and groom. And they were both completely intact with their beautiful bridal costumes in this gorgeous Spanish attire, and as soon as they opened the lid, *poof!* Up they went—just into thin air. I thought as a child that must have been some sight—to see them just disappear like that."

Lorna remembers her father as a very fair and honest businessman who lost everything in the Great Depression. One sunny afternoon this spring, as Lorna and I sat in one of her favorite gardens, she told me the story about the day her father found out he had lost the family fortune. "He and his brothers [who ran the factory] lost millions of dollars in that depression. They had stock in the company and some people who had stocks were jumping from windows and my father, who had lost the most, came home whistling. I was home with my mother and I heard him whistling coming up the walk. I was in the kitchen, I remember, and he said to my mother that he needed to tell her something. They went into the study and I thought what is he going to tell her? He told her that they lost everything, completely everything, and then there was a silence, and my mother said 'Well, that will be fun to start all over again, won't it? Won't that just be great!" For Lorna, it exemplified their wonderful values. They were not attached to the material world, but believed in each other and in their life together.

"He told her that they lost everything, completely everything, and then there was a silence, and my mother said 'Well, that will be fun to start all over again, won't it?'"

Lorna was encouraged from a very early age to explore her creative talents. It happened, Lorna explains, because she was "born into it." Her earliest memory of knowing what she wanted to do in her life came at the age of six, when she learned the alphabet and began to read and write. She soon began to write her own little books as a child about her own life or stories that she made up and to write poetry. It was only a few years later that some of her poems were published in the *Cincinnati Post*.

Her love of writing continued throughout her youth. She became editor of her school newspaper, but during this time she also discovered her love of acting. She would create her own "extemporaneous" plays and perform them for the neighborhood children in her own backyard. As she grew older, she continued to explore and develop both her love of writing and acting, becoming very active in large drama productions while in high school. Graduation from high school meant a major decision: would she study writing or theater? Encouraged by her parents, she opted to study dramatic arts at Tulane University in New Orleans. After her first year at Tulane she decided to focus on studying theater so she went back to Cincinnati to get her university degree in dramatic arts at the University of Cincinnati. It was there that she first studied with John Redhead Froome. This was followed by studies at Columbia University in New York, and finally back home at the Cincinnati College of Music and Dramatic Arts.

After college, she continued to develop her dramatic career, performing with many stock theater companies in New England and New York. She studied the English tradition of acting with John Redhead Froome, who had acted and trained in England with some of the leading actors of that time. Eventually, she went on to win the Midwest Shakespearean Contest for Actors, and returned home to become the founder and director of the Cincinnati Civic Theater. Then around 1940, following her marriage to a Cuban physician whom she met as a student at Tulane University, she moved to Havana, where she lived for nearly eighteen years.

I realize that each time I leave my visit with Lorna, I see more and more of myself in her, and I start to see the reasons for our bond.

On many of my visits Lorna talked about Cuba as though it were the most defining time in her life. One cold winter day when I visit, the sky is threatening rain. Despite the weather or perhaps because of it, she insists on going outside to talk. These are the kinds of risks that Lorna allows herself to take–to feel the fullness of the air, perhaps even a sprinkle or two on her face and with any luck to get caught in a full shower. So we head out to the garden to sit once again, bundled with hats, scarves and coats, catching up on our week. Our friendship seems to have shifted from that of a writer interviewing her subject to one of two friends sharing the latest details of their lives. I realize that each time I leave my visit with Lorna, I see more and more of myself in her, and I start to see the reasons for our bond.

On this day, the leaves had all fallen from the trees and the branches were left to bare their skeletal structures, telling a story of their own about the path of growth each branch had taken over the years. Lorna has been trying to get to the story of her life in Cuba for many visits now and we keep getting sidetracked for one reason or another. But today in the garden, the air heavy with moisture, the time seems right. It's just the two of us sequestered among the bare trees and she begins to tell me about her life in Havana: "When I arrived in the port of Havana for the first time, I was swept away with the smells, feeling the pulse and sounds, and seeing the colors, rich and vibrant, of the Cuban culture. I knew right then that I was home".

So began her love affair with Cuba, which to this day has never been far from her heart.

Lorna and her husband had two children, Kristin and Victor. Both were raised in Havana. It was in Lorna's new home that her career in drama took off. She began working with distinguished Cuban and European actors and playwrights, including the Spaniard José Rubia Barcia. A drama professor who had fled Spain to Cuba in the '30s to escape the Spanish Civil War, Rubia Barcia later became known for his collaboration and friendship with the famous Spanish filmmaker Luis Buñuel. Together, Lorna and Rubia

Barcia formed the Academia de Artes Dramáticas (the Academy of Dramatic Arts) in Havana. Their mission for the academy was to offer the pueblo (people) free training in dramatic arts, taking theater from its traditional hierarchical place to where it could be understood, enjoyed and experienced by all.

Lorna recalls, "I arrived in Cuba when theater was in a very old-fashioned state, following the Spanish way of producing plays; to me, it was incongruous and incredible." Lorna had been trained in the English style of a very disciplined theater, with its studied approach. The Cuban approach was something new to her. She goes on, "They would get a play and read it once with the director and then talk about it a little and then that was the end—they just performed it. They never rehearsed it. And these were very, very fine actors, but it was all so spontaneous. They did not memorize anything... It was funny. It would be like this: while an actor was saying 'Oh my darling don't leave me!' the prompter at the same time is saying to them, 'Now take out a cigarette and turn you're head toward her and smile,' and the audience knew it was happening." Still, she says, "the plays were good. They were very fine Spanish dramatists and playwrights, depending mostly on their personal dramatic instincts and feelings."

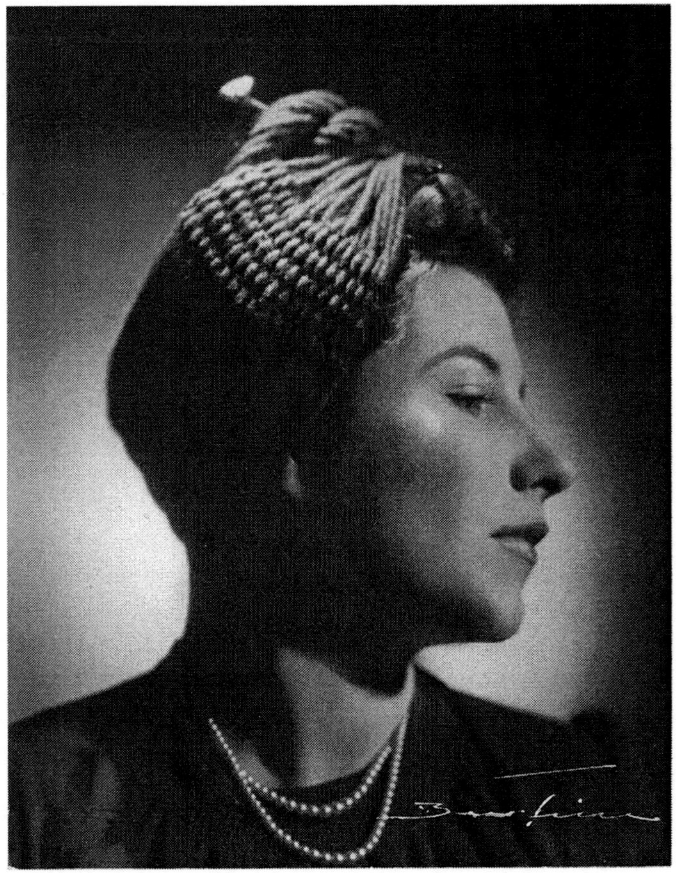

Lorna, the actress, in Cuba

It would be a challenge to change the direction of Cuban theater. It was the 1940s and as a young American woman, Lorna had to prove her strength and ability to lead her actors through this transformation. "One of the leading actors of the time came from Spain to Cuba to work in the production. Everyone said that it was impossible, that you cannot

"I had to make my own way, as a woman, but my work seemed to get me in."

make him learn a line. That he just wouldn't do that. And I was only a critter of twenty-eight or so and many of the actors [mostly men] were older than I, and very attractive people with a lot of pride in their craft. "

One particular account personifies Lorna's determined spirit and what she was up against, both as a dramatist and a woman. Four famous male Spanish actors were playing poker in the back of the theater while Lorna was rehearsing for an upcoming play. Students from the Academia lined both sides of the theater as they watched the rehearsal. Lorna recounts, "It came time for the cue of these actors and their cue was called and they kept playing and paid no attention–just kept playing poker. I called and said 'Carlos and Enrique and Otto, your cue is coming up in about one minute and nothing happened, no response. Then I said 'Your cue is here', and they did nothing still and so I stopped the rehearsal. Everybody was watching to see what was going to happen, all eyes were on me and it was one of those moments, you know? And I came down from the stage and I marched over to their table and I said 'You have missed your cue!' and I threw up their table... and their hands were white knuckled like you could see they were not sure what to do. I just stood there waiting to see what was going to happen. I did not know whether they were going to punch me or not and then one of them said, 'We will go up.'"

"And they left the table—just left the whole thing with the money and cards and all, all over the place, and went up to rehearse. It was a big moment for me you know: the challenge and the battle between two ideologies. I had to make my own way, as a woman, but my work seemed to get me in."

Lorna is also proud of how the famous academy she helped found attracted students from the pueblo. I started to see how what she did in Cuba created great changes in a world where so many were not given the opportunity to explore the creative arts. "There was an young sailor who was scrubbing the floors of his admiral's swimming pool and he had his bucket sitting on top of the newspaper, open to the page where we had placed an ad for the Academia. The ad said that we were looking for people who where interested in pursuing the dramatic arts and that we had full scholarships for those who applied," she recalls. When the young man saw the ad, he left his pail and brush and went immediately to Havana to enroll in the Academia. The student later went on to become one of the great talents to come out of our program."

She goes on to recount a similar incident: "There was another man—the same thing—he was a country farmer out milking his cow one morning, and [he] saw the ad in the paper. And don't you know, he also left the cow and the pail full of milk and came to Havana to study with us!" Her accounts testify to how Lorna profoundly touched the culture of the Cuban people.

Her accounts testify to how Lorna profoundly touched the culture of the Cuban people.

From the Academia de Artes Dramáticas emerged the Patronato del Teatro, Theatralia, which produced both native and international theater pieces. For the first time, Cuba became the stage for worldwide theater—from Chekhov and Sartre to Maugham and Lope de Vega. Lorna had found her place in the world. It was an electrifying time in her life. She wrote, produced and directed, as well as acted, and was one of the driving forces that helped to establish a new love of theater in Havana. During her time in Havana, Lorna was honored for her commitment and dedication to Cuban culture with her induction into the Order of José Martí (Orden José Martí). The prestigious award is given in memory of the famous nineteenth-century Cuban poet and revolutionary José Martí.

With the flourishing of theater, Lorna was appointed by the Cuban government to produce and direct National Dramatic Festivals in Cuba. It was at one of these festivals that she met Felix Guerrero, one of Cuba's leading musicians and composers at the time. The encounter began a long and mutual admiration for each other's work and life.

On one of my visits, I find Lorna in the library, researching on the Internet with the help of one of her caregivers. She had been looking for information on her old friend Felix, tracking his music and the details of his career. Lorna informs me that she has finally tracked him down. She looks flustered so I ask her if everything is okay. She tells me that she has just learned he had died a few years ago. "We have been on this thing so long looking for traces of him, but nothing about when he died or the circumstances. So finally Martha [her caregiver] and I resorted to a newspaper and we found an article that was written in Cuban. It was written in such beautiful Cuban Spanish in the old style of language and it made me so homesick. And I contacted the writer and he was excited about hearing from me. But this was a very cold way to find out about his [Felix's] death, very cold."

As usual, Lorna seeks refuge and comfort in nature. She tells me she wants to go outside to smell the air, and let it fill her lungs with open space. We venture out into the garden again. It is a dark day, but there is a rainbow in the middle of a dark cloud with the promise of sunlight. The sun is fighting to break through, and suddenly a few bright rays begin to shine. It reminds both of us of the winter skies of a Turner painting, a symbol of hope.

Lorna has been devastated by Felix's death. Despite her efforts to write about him, she feels stuck. It is just too deep a thing right now, she says. It is now mid- February, the air has unseasonably warmed, and everything is in bloom. Lorna asks that I ring an outdoor chime for her so that she can hear its sound, and then she takes me to a part of the garden with a fig tree that is brimming over with its ripe fruit. I pick some figs for us to eat. Lorna says she used to hate these false springs, but now she loves them. They are a chance to see the burst of color and a way to light up the darkness of the rainy Bay Area winters—a chance to relieve another sorrow added to her heart.

She then begins to tell me about when she left Cuba after eighteen years. It was in the late 1950s. Her children were getting older and they needed to see what life was like in other places. So with great regret and sadness, she realized it was time to leave Havana and bring her children back home to the United States. In an article written for the Havana press, entitled "The Arrival and Departure of Lorna De Sosa," one of the actors that she had worked with at the Academia was quoted as saying that Lorna had "changed the whole taste of modern theatre in Cuba." To have made this kind of an impact is a testament to the tenacity, vision and the success of Lorna's life endeavors in Cuba.

Lorna left a piece of her heart in Cuba, but her departure led to a new phase of her life. After she arrived back in the United States, things started to boom even more in her career. Playwright Antonio Bueno Vallejo, one of Spain's leading intellectuals who was widely considered to be the father of Spanish modern theater, granted Lorna exclusive rights to produce his works in America. Her career grew to international proportions when she was later appointed as the representative for Latin America in the International Theater Institute, headquartered in Paris. She continued to live around the world, including, Zurich, where she studied at the Jungian Institute, Greece and Italy for a short time.

It is now spring. The winter has brought us torrents of rain, but the weather is improving. On many of my visits to Lorna during the winter we had been bound up inside. Today when I arrive, Lorna is itching to get outside right away. She is in true form and ready to tell me some stories. Lorna is armed with her cell phone and on our way out to the garden, she chats with an old friend. "I was in between two worlds when you called earlier, so to speak, going in between the old ladies home to the front common room where there was a crazy hat party going on... and my phone went dead and that is why you suddenly disappeared from my ear. I will call you back later. Love you. Bye-bye." Phone now neatly tucked away in her bag, she inhales deeply and whispers her mantra, "Hello, world," as we roll down the garden path to her favorite bench.

And so when Lorna begins to talk, I enter her world and relive a memory of my own about a time when life seemed so idyllic.

As I wait for our conversation to begin, I am reminded of a time when I sat with my grandmother on a bench outside on a sunny spring day. I remember being hypnotized by the cadence of her voice—the drifting remnants of her Irish brogue rising and falling as she emphasized certain phrases. In these stories, she would weave a scene, and I would watch my own cultural history unfold before me—seeing in my mind images of what people looked like and seeing the green of the grass and the blue of the ocean that she described. I have always loved to hear stories, especially those told firsthand. And so when Lorna begins to talk, I enter her world and relive a memory of my own about a time when life seemed so idyllic.

At ninety-two, Lorna's memory is remarkably clear and as she begins, I see the details of her story as if it were my own. She begins to recount the effect of an extraordinary historic event, perhaps her most unforgettable moment, which also had been etched in my much younger memory. Her children now grown, Lorna settled in New York for a time, but often visited Washington, D.C., where her son was living. John F. Kennedy was now in office and while spending time in the nation's capitol, Lorna was shocked to discover how unaware this city's international population was of Latin American culture. Lorna knew of the Kennedy's interest in Latin America, so she came up with an idea for a program that would help to increase awareness of Latin cultures in Washington. It was to be sponsored with the United Nations in which each embassy would support a month of cultural events. "We would have the art, dance and performances [from that country], theater in English and Spanish and whatever cultural thing they wanted to offer... So I was going to have an interview with both JFK and Jackie right after they were to return from Texas. They were very interested in the idea."

I knew where this was going to end. My memory of the Kennedy assassination is a sharp one that will forever be engraved in my mind as one of the most seminal events of my childhood. I was five years old and in kindergarten. We were dismissed early and everyone was crying—my teachers, the parents of children picking up their kids from school. I remember my mother pulling up in our station wagon and when I got in the car she was crying. At home, my father and neighbors were glued to the TV in our living room, watching cars racing down the streets of Dallas. Then a few days later our family and neighbors gathered around our TV once again, weeping as the horse-drawn carriage carried Kennedy's body through the streets of Washington with the crowds waving for the last time. The crying continued for what seemed like days. It was a time of eternal sadness, it seemed to my young mind, which came over my house like a dark cloud that would never clear.

"He was so wonderful and there was just a tremendous kind of energy that he gave this country and a buoyancy and we just knew everything was going to be fine. You know?"

I asked Lorna what is was like for her when Kennedy was shot?

"Oh, it was one of the great tragedies of this country and of my own personal life because, I loved him so... I hadn't any interest in politics for many years. But when I heard Kennedy—oh, just my whole being was moved. And that happened to everyone. It was a shock wave. He was so wonderful and there was just a tremendous kind of energy that he gave this country and a buoyancy and we just knew everything was going to be fine. You know?"

Lorna continued: "You had to see the way people walked in the streets in New York and Washington, as if there were a lightness in their steps and they were interested in things, all kinds of things. When he got shot, I was right by St. Patrick's Cathedral in New York. I was actually going right across the street to Saks to get something fabulous to wear for the meeting with the Kennedy's and I heard someone say something about the president being shot. I turned and I said 'That isn't funny to make jokes about things like that'. And this man said, 'It isn't a joke, ma'am.'"

Lorna describes how an announcement was made that the president had been shot, but was still alive. What struck her, she says, is that "suddenly there was no class-consciousness of any kind. We were all just human beings in pain—and I was standing there and they had put a huge portrait of JFK up outside the cathedral. There was a very elegant women—oh, so bejeweled and she had on a beautiful fur coat and she stood there and there was a little black boy and he came up and he started crying."

Lorna is struggling to keep her composure. These feelings still live so deeply inside of her. She tells me it's sad to remember, and then, as I had seen her do before, she scolds herself, "Oh Lorna, now behave—now just stop it." But she explains that it's not just sorrow she feels, but the beauty of what came out of that day for her. "It's half and half [half sorrow and half beauty] is why I am tearful about it."

Lorna is a dyed-in-the-wool Democrat, passionate about politics and political history.

She continues: "This boy stood there and that woman put her arms around him and they hugged each other and they were standing there, holding each other and crying... I walked away [after the announcement of Kennedy's death] in a daze and I crossed over the street and there was a very fancy car with a chauffeur in the front of a building. And a woman was sitting in the back seat and I was in such a daze I just didn't care. I walked up to the car; I opened the door without asking and got into the car. And the women said 'Oh my dear' and we hugged and cried together."

Weeks after Kennedy's death, the power of the event continued. One day when Lorna was sitting in a coffee shop off of Fifth Avenue, a workman with a hardhat sat down next to her at the counter. She recounts every detail: "He ordered pie and coffee. Well it came, and he suddenly pushed it away and burst into tears—this big muscle guy, you know. And he said 'Oh excuse me' or something and he was just sitting there crying. And I said 'I know what you are crying about.' And he said, 'Yes, you do.' And we sat there and held hands. And that happened in trains and in buses, everywhere. People would suddenly start to cry."

Lorna is a dyed-in-the-wool Democrat, passionate about politics and political history. She admits being blind to any criticisms of either Kennedy or Clinton. "I don't give a rat what they have done with their personal lives," she tells me, "because we did not bring them into office for their personal lives." She attributes the country's disillusionment and cynicism to Nixon. "To see what Nixon and the whole bunch did was a great shattering blow to this country. We have had all kinds of shattering blows since then."

Lorna chuckles as she remembers a moment that illustrated her political passion, during the Kennedy-Nixon presidential debates. "I was so wound up I was barely breathing. And just in the midst of that someone called me and I automatically picked up the phone and they said, 'Hello Lorna?' and I said, 'How dare you! Listen to the debate!' and I hung up!" We both start to laugh and it feels good. It breaks that sadness we were locked into remembering and we both feel light again.

Lorna continued to live between New York and California with short stints in Europe until eventually she landed in Berkeley and made it her permanent home. She lived in Berkeley for thirty-five years before her arrival at the Salem Lutheran Home. During those years, Lorna continued to lead a rich creative life, but directed her efforts away from the dramatic arts and focused on her other life-long passion—writing. She continued to write poetry and work on a manuscript for a novel based on the period when she lived in Cuba.

During this time, she taught applied theology at the Graduate Theological Union in Berkeley. Here she worked with men and women from all walks of life that had given up their previous professions to volunteer in churches around the country. Her background as a director in the dramatic arts was a perfect match to help these new volunteers learn how to express themselves and work from their hearts in their service to the church. She also taught dramatic arts for a short time at San Francisco State University and acted as director in the lector-training program of lay people at St. Albert's Priory, a house of studies for the Western Province of the Dominican order in Oakland.

But what she talks about most from this era is the beautiful Spanish-style apartment building on Spruce Street where she enjoyed a sweeping view of the San Francisco Bay from her living room window. It's a view that she misses dearly—of the water and the big open sky, the fog rolling in over Mt. Tamalpais and San Francisco and then crossing over the Bay to creep its way up into the hills. On clear days she could see all three bridges—the Golden Gate, the Bay Bridge and the Richmond Bridge—as well as a clear shot to Angel Island and the perfect view of the beautiful skyline of San Francisco.

One sunny day when I visit Lorna this spring, her old neighbor Bill also stops by for a visit. He and Lorna started to reminisce about the old apartment building where they met as neighbors and where Bill still lives. Lorna's apartment was so big, says Bill, that she was "like a marble rattling around in it." I thought of Lorna with all this open space around her inside the apartment and the exterior space through her windows. I think of how hard it has been for her to make a home in the room she currently shares with her roommate, Teena. She has been trying to stuff a life's worth of belongings into half of a small area. At times during my visits to her, we were consumed with talking about where or how to store her belongings. These are the artifacts that have helped to keep her memory so sharp. They are the threads to a life that has been well lived—photographs, books on art, history, poetry and literature, art that once adorned her home, manuscripts of her writings, and letters that she has saved from friends and family. They are the objects that she looked at every day for many years of her life, that traveled with her through all of her adventures. These are what make her room at Salem Lutheran her home.

As Lorna, Bill and I walk to the garden, the trees are in full bloom and bursting with color. "Oh, look, the trees are suddenly getting all dressed up again!" Lorna cries. As we sit in the garden, she talks about her life as it is now. She begins to tell me about her roommate Teena, a former librarian and highly educated woman who now spends most of her day sleeping. During the times when I have visited with Lorna, Teena has always seemed withdrawn from life. While awake, Teena tries to communicate by yelling and screaming—not any words, but just by making loud sounds. Lorna has grown to understand something about Teena that most people don't see. Teena, Lorna says, is trying in her own way to reach outside of her world to the people around her in the only way she is able to. "I make her see pictures by talking to her from across the room. I tell her what the weather is like outside and that the tree outside our window has

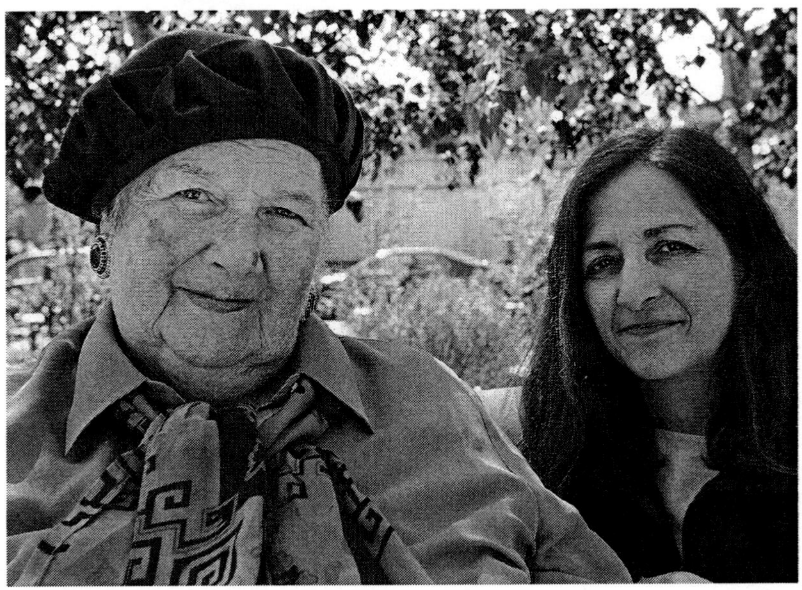

Lorna with her writer, Trena

Though most of the nursing staff says Teena cannot hear or understand, Lorna persists in believing that some part of her roommate is still present and trying to find a way to communicate.

new leaves and what color they are."

Though most of the nursing staff says Teena cannot hear or understand, Lorna persists in believing that some part of her roommate is still present and trying to find a way to communicate. She started to pay close attention to Teena's sounds and realized that when she talked to Teena about the world outside, Teena would become quiet and peaceful, as though she were hanging on to Lorna's words. One night, when Teena was really struggling, Lorna sang her name "Teena, Teena, Teena." Lorna's sweet voice helped to calm Teena. "That's when I knew she was listening," says Lorna. "So when I was talking on the phone and Teena was making her noises I would just say 'Teena, I am trying to talk on the phone, but I can't hear because you are talking too loud. Please talk lower. Would you do that for me?' And she would stop." Lorna talks to Teena now daily. As they are going to sleep, Lorna will say. "Thank you Teena. You are so nice. There is a little angel on your pillow so you will have sweet dreams." And Teena will fall quietly asleep.

Lorna tells me that she believes in doing what you can for others, even if it seems like you might not get anywhere. As she leaves her room to go out into the garden with me, she peeks through the curtain into Teena's side of the room, and says softly, "I am going out now Teena. It's a nice spring day. The sky is blue and the flowers are blooming." Lorna admits that she would very happy if she knew that some of the images she describes for Teena really got into her head to help her dream of the world she once engaged with.

Though Lorna maintains an upbeat attitude, she struggles with macular degeneration that has seriously limited her ability to read. She also had a serious fall while still living in her apartment in Berkeley, and arthritis now makes it impossible for her to walk. But she continues to use her creativity in a way that doesn't require her eyes or legs. At the age of ninety, she published a book of poems, entitled *Who Turned the Grass On?* One of her poems, "Quiet Song" seems to address her later years:

Quiet Song

5 a.m.
I am awake.
The words I have been searching for,
the rhythm, the form
have come in half-sleep.
Like butterflies, they will escape
at my finger's edge, if I am not swift.
I hurry to the desk with wonderful intensity,
thinking about the great events
of the heart and of the cities,
and the words have not escaped.
                    Pain. I had forgotten.
                    Arthritis, is that my new master?
As I am about to rise from the desk
in this foggy predawn,
the bird in a very small voice
quietly begins a song.
A small quiet song
from the dark.
                    Is this now what I must sing?

In April while visiting Lorna, I bring along the Nine Lives project coordinator for her to meet. While talking about living in Berkeley, we realize in an amazing coincidence that another elder in this book, Helen Rand Parish, is an old friend of Lorna's. The two lived right down the street from each other and now live in nursing homes separated by a ten-minute ride. They had been out of touch for years. Lorna often thought of Helen and wondered where she was and if they would ever meet again. Upon realizing this discovery, Lorna rolls her wheelchair away from where we are sitting, puts her face in her hands and begins to weep, joyful with the news that her friend is still alive. Despite our best intentions to unite the two friends, Helen's heath declines rapidly in the few weeks following and sadly Lorna is never able to meet with her dear friend again.

Lorna wheels closer to me and lays her hand on mine. "You look tired." She says. "I am," I reply.

The day I hear of Helen's passing, I feel Lorna's pain. How would I tell her? I call her and she tells me that she has already heard the news. She is saddened by the loss and the missed chance to see Helen one last time. We make plans to see each other and a few days later I make a visit.

This has been a hard month for both of us, she having suffered yet another loss of a friend and me having worked around the clock, fighting to meet a publication deadline for a journal I edit. We decide to sit outside in the garden to soak up some of the warm sunshine to boost our spirits. We move out to the path that leads up to the garden where the Mexican table and chair set is—the one with the big blossoming roses carved into the wood. I sit in one of the chairs, feeling like I could sink into the largeness of it. I lay my hand on the arm of the chair and outline one of the carved roses with my finger. Lorna wheels closer to me and lays her hand on mine. "You look tired." She says. "I am," I reply.

I am teetering on the brink of exhaustion and I am not sure whether to laugh or cry. We talk for a while—just to catch up. It's been a few weeks since we have met face to face and I realize that I have missed her. The sun is warm and feels good—rejuvenating. I need to sit in this garden, the same way Lorna does. But the sun is now setting in the sky and it is time for me to go home. We hug and kiss each other's cheeks and say our good-byes. As I turn to walk toward my car, Lorna calls to me. I turn back to her and she says, "Be good to yourself, take care and do something that will make you feel good." I tell her I will, and as I turn to walk away from her sitting in the garden, my heart aches. I realize that we have come to know each other deeply. Not that we know everything about the details of our days, but that we have come to know each other's heart. As I walk away, I know that I have found a friend. ■

Our thanks to Lorna De Sosa for allowing us to reprint "Quiet Song," from her book Who Turned the Grass On? (Small Poetry Press, Concord CA, 2003).

WRITER'S PROFILE

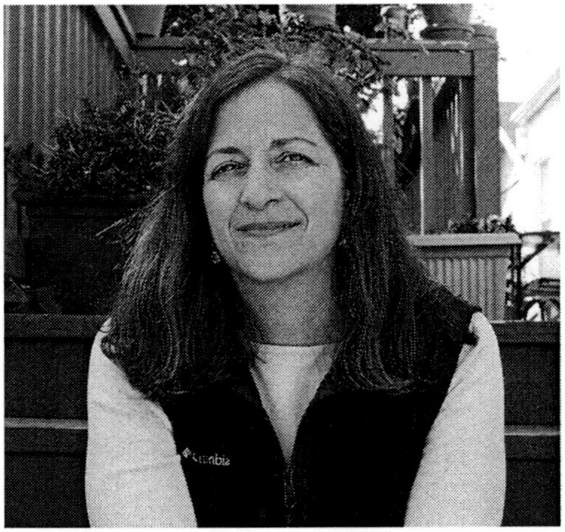

Trena Noval

When I was in my early twenties, my grandmother was placed in a nursing home. My grandfather had passed away and my parents were not equipped with the tools or the skills to take care of my grandmother's declining health. It was a very difficult decision for my mother to make and both of my parents labored over it for quite some time. They wanted the best quality of life for my grandmother, so they searched for a home that they thought would be the best place for her. It was a very painful transition for my grandmother. Typical of her generation, she had taken care of her parents and I don't think she could understand why my parents had made the decision they had about her life.

For Lorna, too, it is difficult living in a nursing home. It is not her preferred place to live out her days—but she understands why she is there, despite her longing for her previous life. It is really her cheerful disposition, tenacity and ability to stay networked with her community through her total embrace of modern technologies that have been an inspiration to me. It has been a privilege and an honor to be part of this project and to be able to become friends with Lorna.

I am a writer who has primarily written for arts journals and I am more recently a contributing editor of an arts journal based in San Francisco. But I am mainly interested in writing essays and creative non-fiction about experiences that have touched my life. I have always been easily seduced by the spell of a good storyteller. I have a natural curiosity and interest in people's lives and how experiences get played out. Our culture does not pay enough attention to the stories and lessons of our elder population. That is why the *Nine Lives* project has been a gift to me—of listening to amazing stories, of remembering my own life markers and contributing to a monument of sorts about a history worth knowing.

MILDRED HARRIS

Willow Tree Nursing Center
Oakland, California
with
Cleavon Smith

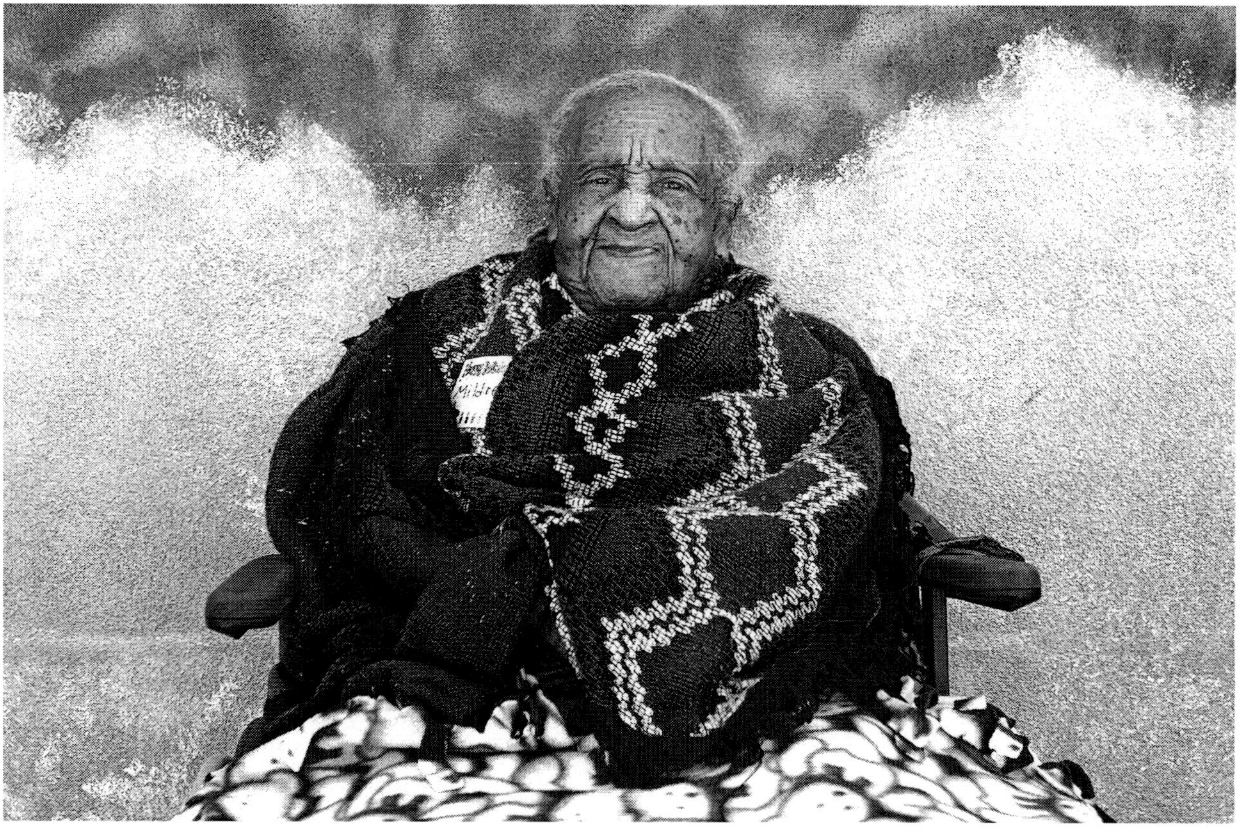

"What you give from love is no small thing at all"

"Mister," she calls me Mister, sometimes "child," "brother-man." This time she calls me Mister. "Mister, I thank God that my mother and father passed before they ended up in a place like this. Do you know the truth when you hear it? Glad to my heart my mother and father were gone before they hit a place like this." Over the rail of her bed, she pokes her right forefinger, the skin wrinkled and spotted with age, but the conviction in her point is punctuated nonetheless. She means here, Willow Tree Nursing Center in Oakland. She points to the ceiling. I squint, trying to keep from crying myself, not really wanting to comprehend what she means, not wanting to think she has any sense of a better life outside the nursing home. Mildred is ninety-nine years old in exactly one month, and her wits are with her. She knows what she says and means it. Desperately.

Mildred is ninety-nine years old in exactly one month, and her wits are with her. She knows what she says and means it. Desperately.

I could tell you facts. Mildred did...or Mildred wishes she had done... The population of Tallulah in 1909 was...or the population of Tallulah was no greater than...Mildred graduated from...or Mildred never graduated from...

I could also give you an arc of time. On April 19, 1906... In the summer of 1932... After an early spring shower in 1995...

But I can't find a discernable beginning to her story. There were groves of pecan trees; there was a two-story barn; there was God. It is possible when all these met, Mildred's story began. It is possible. More likely under the urge of all things meeting, we may find the beginnings of her beginning. Supposedly, according to myth and legend, according to math and literature, according to the smile on Mildred's face, it begins in beauty.

But the first time I saw Mildred cry, I made a great mistake in interpreting her life. I began her story with pain. I equated her life to the sum of her tears. I reduced the tales of her childhood and motherhood as anecdotal. I was sad for Mildred and felt sorry for the fact that her life had come to this point where she could only give me a glimpse of the past, a time and a person long gone by. And if Mildred wanted to prove to me that she was more than just a woman of memories, more than just a subject of a story to be submitted in some book, she had hard work cut out for her, but hard work was no stranger to Mildred. Soon I would learn. Soon I would see who Mildred *is*.

"My mother didn't pay attention to the clock; she just go on by the rooster. She would call us in the morning, 'Children, the rooster, he calling.'"

"From Can to Can't, that's when we worked." Mildred has the tendency to lean towards you when she's punctuating her points. Eventually I will hear her tell me this expression several times, but the first time she tells me the hours of her workdays on her family's farm in Tallulah, Louisiana I'm being introduced to her. A Lutheran chaplain who sends Mildred a card if she misses her weekly visit with Mildred, the executive director of ELDERGIVERS, and I are all standing around her bed. Her head swings to each of us surrounding her. We can tell by the way she takes the time to look each of us in our eyes it is important that we understand her words, which are sometimes difficult to hear, especially in the late afternoon hours. But just as important, I learn in time, is that we understand the woman whose image these words paint.

"We had a fireplace and on the mantel was a big ol' clock with big ol' hands, big as my hand." She raises her hand to show me. "My mother didn't pay attention to the clock; she just go on by the rooster. She would call us in the morning, 'Children, the rooster, he calling.' I used to tell my sister, 'Listen to that big ol' loud-mouthed rooster."

She has the power to transform herself through sharing her memories, and I see a somewhere-near-nine-year-old girl curled in her bed making the same faces she's making at me, squinted eyes and pursed, pouting lips, wishing not hear her call to work. For the sake of clarity she mocks the call of the rooster, "Who, who, whooooo." We laugh together at the sound of the rooster's call, the little girl dreading the call, and the woman making the call in the bed next to me. Mildred turns her head from me towards the ceiling and sounds the call again. As the last note echoes in the corners of the room and in our minds, she turns to me and we share another lingering smile.

Her days on her family's farm near the Mississippi River, were filled with work and service, the two never apart from one another. "Ever since I was big enough to carry a bucket across a field, I was trained to help people." From what I gathered, I wouldn't say it was as much of a training her parents provided her as it was a modeling, and what she learned from her parents, over the years she grew to appreciate and was proud of. It was something she too would pass on to her son and share with me.

Blue was a large plot of land, several dozens of acres. "Me and Ruby would look out the second story of the barn and all you could see was our papa's." Located near the Mississippi River two dozen miles from Vicksburg, Mississippi, Blue had all the fixings one could expect on a good, productive farm—corn, cotton, cucumber, watermelon, rivercane, sugarcane (you could use those two for syrup), mushmelons and more. "You name it," Mildred tells me once she tires of making her list. "Wild ducks running around...hogs all around. You name it." She looks to me intently. Lips and cheeks like one trying to whistle by sucking air in, her eyes the color of polished pecans staring through me, she holds this expression not, as I've learned, waiting for my reply, but because her sight is leaving her.

Her face lights up; her shoulders bounce; she swivels her head back and forth when taking a deep breath; she shakes her fingers and squeezes them when counting down the details.

Her home was a place to engage all of the senses. Of the butter they would churn from the milk of her father's cows she says, "Mister, if you tasted it, you wouldn't believe how good butter could be." On their "big, long porch" her mother kept "flower pots with every color growing from 'em," and stepping down from the back door the family would walk into her mother's flower garden "with all kinds of flowers, honeysuckle, morning glories, roses..." Mildred sprinkles the scene with her fingers running in the air over different parts of her body lying in her bed.

It's hard to keep up with Mildred once she starts talking about her family's farm in Louisiana. Her face lights up; her shoulders bounce; she swivels her head back and forth when taking a deep breath; she shakes her fingers and squeezes them when counting down the details. Even though she spent less than a quarter of her life in Louisiana, it's obvious that Tallulah is where she calls home.

"Papa had a big barn. Stall on the first floor, a cornhouse too. There was a trough with grain. Mules and horses and when it got cold, cows could go in and eat when they get ready. There was hay over the trough. He kept potatoes right behind the corn crib." Not being a farm boy, I have a hard time digesting the images. Just when I begin a mental picture, she continues on. There's an excitement in her body; it's contagious, and I could care less for the exact picture of the barn than I care for the moment she's sharing. "He had a smokehouse as big as this section in the room. From there to this here over here." I try my best to trace what she has pointed to. There's a door that has a photocopied photograph of Mildred's grandparents and parents as well as a photograph of Mildred when she was around seventy-five-years-old. In the photo she has a full head of hair

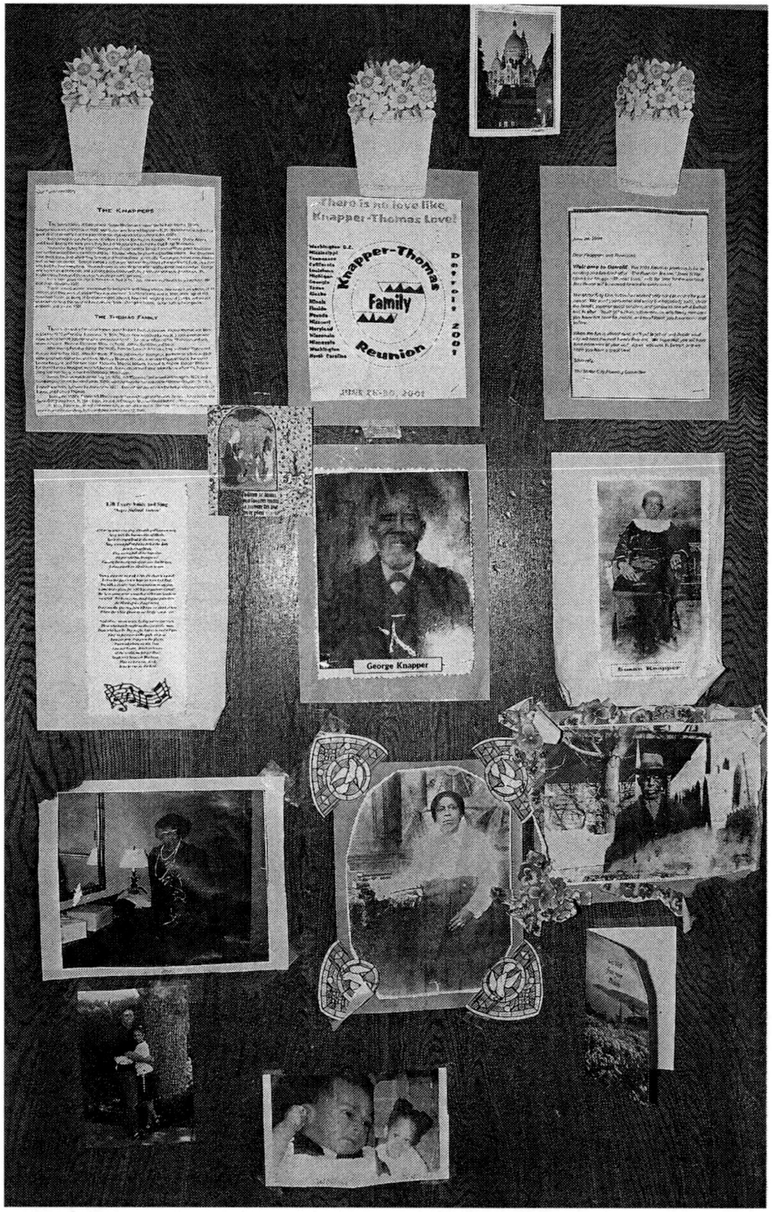

The door in Mildred's room

salted, with some gray. She's wearing a maroon dress with a flower on her lapel. She's obviously posing, nothing exaggerated except the pause anticipating the photographers pressing the button. From the door I trace the width of this smokehouse following her point to the sliding glass door five feet over. I expand my approximation a few feet in width and length. The smokehouse she describes with the strain of her voice and the unwrinkling of her face is big. The room where she has spent the last ten years of her life is small; no "section" of it can contain the smokehouse she is describing. "We had it all in there—fish, beef, pork."

In many parts of the country, especially the rural South, people consider where a person is from to be indicative of who a person is. The expression "Don't forget where you come from" is synonymous with "Don't forget who you are." I'm reminded of this as I listen to Mildred's story, as she does her work on me. The key to her trick, how she works on me, is her apparent love of her home. When she begins shuffling in bed to tell me about life on her family's farm, failing sight or not, she can see me edge my way towards her. She begins to see a reflection of herself in my eyes replacing that nearly translucent image of her I had. As I begin to recognize how these moments she shares with me reveal who she is, not who she was, the true Mildred assumes her rightful place before me and the less-than-Mildred-idea seeps into the forgotten corners of the nursing home along with the fading notes of music hardly heard from the staff's break room.

In many parts of the country, especially the rural South, people consider where a person is from to be indicative of who a person is.

The more I get to know Mildred, who she is, where she's from, the more comfortable I become with my visits to Willow Tree in East Oakland, Mildred's home for the past ten years. I begin to slide though the doors at Willow Tree recognizing the familiar faces of the residents I pass. I notice the staff's laughter doesn't end in the break room or the hallways; it's carried with each worker into the rooms of the residents they serve. I lightly step to Mildred's door so as not to disturb anyone and find her awake. It takes her a second to see me or maybe she waits until she can see some form of her real self in my eyes. This takes a couple of seconds because seeing Mildred lying in her bed, her eyes closed, her chest hardly moving, I focus on death. Or perhaps I get stuck on the possibility that I will relieve Mildred of her post in only a matter of time. Regardless, the result of all my fears is seeing Mildred as a nursing home resident rather than a beautiful ninety-nine-year-old woman whose entire being could outshine the light of the Colossus a thousand times.

It takes a while. I'm a work in progress. But work is nothing from which Mildred has ever shied away.

She looks at me, the corner of her lips poised for a smile that bursts into a laugh carrying through her entire body ending with a clap, when she sees me smile. These are the stories I have begun to look forward to. At first I could articulate how I was enjoying getting to know Mildred as a child; eventually I came to understand how I was beginning to see the Mildred I met at Willow Tree as the child of that child.

"Ohh..." Some things almost lift Mildred out of her bed. If she can't take me to her home in Louisiana, she will bring it to me. Her body is the home she is speaking of. She rises to lift it before me to see in its fullness. "All the time people asking for something. 'Rosie, can I have a slice o' ham?' And she just give it to 'em. Never said no."

Her mother, Rosina, was a giving person. Mildred, making her somewhere-near-nine-years-old faces, shares with me how her mother took care of the people throughout their community. "Didn't care who you were. Everyday. Breakfast...dinner...supper. Every one of them meals she fixed their food and took care of others, and she'd send Mildred (here she nods her head at me to remind me how her mother's service put Mildred to work) to "take it to 'em with grease on her legs and a pleasant face on." She ends her sentence nodding to the cadence of her words. Obviously that's a saying she heard much as a child.

Later, when compiling my notes, I realized why her mother made sure Mildred was presentable when she took food to others.

For Christmas I took cookies to Mildred. Nothing special. I told her how it was just a little something for her for the holidays. She replied, "What you give from love is no small thing at all." By making Mildred grease her legs and put on a good face, Mildred's mother made sure the gifts would be accepted as gifts of neighborly love rather than charity. Over and over Mildred tells me how her mother gave so much to others. In those quiet moments as I recorded the roots of Mildred's personality in my notebook, Mildred would smack her tongue against the roof of her mouth and quickly shift the story to her mother. "I got that from my mother. If anybody was sick they stay with us."

By making Mildred grease her legs and put on a good face, Mildred's mother made sure the gifts would be accepted as gifts of neighborly love rather than charity.

And what Mildred received from her mother, Mildred also returned to her mother. While Mildred was living in Oakland taking care of three other people herself, riding the local buses from one home to another seven days a week, she would return to Louisiana whenever her parents called and told her they needed her. She tells me matter-of-factly, "If they called me and told me they was sick...I was gone." Her voice, frail sometimes in the late afternoon when I usually make my visits, still has the characteristics of the great singer she is. She pushes the "gone" of her last sentence from her diaphragm and curls it in her throat so that I can get the point.

"Everybody was so loved. You knew everybody around and everybody shared whatever they had with each other."

Her mother didn't have a monopoly of this spirit. Several times Mildred tells me how her father, Matt, shared with others. "He's a good ol' man. The men would be out around and tell each other stories, and they'd ask him for seed. He was always trying the newest seeds; when they first come out, my father he had some to share. I remember when he got them Puerto Rican yams. People were high on them. And they'd ask if they could have whatever he had it in him to share." Mildred hesitates. Am I hearing her, listening to her? "And he could always spare a lot. Enough for most people to do what they need. 'Matt, give me just a handful.' He just supplied them."

How did I get from telling how Mildred's days were filled with work and service (the two of them not far apart from each other) to all of the examples of giving? I think because as I got to know Mildred's parents through her tales, how much they had and to what ends they spent the fruits of their labor, I came to understand her family worked so that they could provide not just for the immediate family but also for anyone else in any kind of need. There was a sense in Mildred's tale that where she came from, who she was was a community in which everyone knew very well how much they needed each other.

For weeks I thought I had made a great discovery, synthesizing details that seemed could only be related after great critical inquiry. Then when I started going through my notes I found this quote, "Everybody was so loved. You knew everybody around and everybody shared whatever they had with each other." Then another quote, "Sunday came. Go to church. Laugh and talk. Boy, we was just glad to go to things and give people stuff. All us kids." In light of this, her parents were no different from any other. People worked hard because their survival depended upon their work and the generosity of others. That's just where Mildred is from. Work and service. Work/service.

It would be too idyllic, unfair, dishonest to tell all of this without sharing that Mildred had her complaints. "Listen to that ol' big mouth rooster." Her family was like all the others, but it was also unlike many others. Work and service were connected, but for Mildred and her sisters and brothers on Blue, work was only interrupted by the noon bell and the hours between Can't and Can. "We would get so angry sometimes," Mildred shows me her anger by squinting her eyes and bulging her lips. "Everyone else going to picnic and getting dressed up, but we would be out working."

"We didn't have time out to be free or nothing. Just work, work. Chickens, turkeys, and those stupid goats."

"We didn't have time out to be free or nothing. Just work, work. Chickens, turkeys, and those stupid goats." She pushes her lips even tighter together and further out, making it obvious through her body language that she is sharing a sense of what she really means, who she really is, where she's from. I used to see my daddy make that face at me when he was poking fun and mocking my pouting. My niece has this habit when she doesn't get her way. Mildred has opened to me in this way, telling me more than words, showing me who she is.

It's funny this relationship between facts and what our minds accept or remember. Just like the heavens are capable of holding blue skies and black clouds in the same moment, giving us rain and crisp views, so can a ninety-nine-year-old woman tell contradicting details of her life without contradicting herself. And on those rainy/sunny days a rainbow appears full-arched or maybe one above the other, and we relieve ourselves of our need to remember the days as either sunny or rainy, only finding ourselves mindful of our wonder of the miracle that can't be reduced to a simple dance of light with droplets of water. And for Mildred, with her recollections of harsh days of never-ending work on Blue, with her lips parting, the corners of her mouth stretching, reaching, lifting towards her eyes; a memory hiccups in her throat, and she tells me, "All that work; we was just as happy." She pouts and laughs. She grimaces and smiles. All that work and happy. No time out to be free, and the stories of playing with friends or spending hours in the barn with her sister Ruby.

There was time out. On Sundays mostly. Mildred and the rest of her family along with the world around them were free to worship and spend time together. "A whole lot of us stay after church and talk and some go to each other houses." Some things Mildred tells tilting her head towards you so as to stress the truth of her words, the necessity that you understand. But this she tells me shrugging her shoulders and turning her palms upwards as if to suggest "What else were we to do? We were community." Words echo. "Everybody was so loved...share whatever they had with each other." She continues. "Children enjoyed playing together; going places together, talking together." She adds, "We used to go 'a piece o' the way.'" Saying "a piece o' the way" makes her laugh. It's an old expression she hasn't used except in talking about the old days since she was a young woman in Tallulah. She explains that "a piece o' the way" was how a guest was sent home. The host would walk half-way with the guest allowing both to enjoy each other's company that much longer. Sometimes they would play tag and the guest would walk a piece o' the way back with the host and back again. She smiles. A rainbow.

Before Mildred left for Oakland, the farthest she had ever traveled was to New Orleans. Her family would also sometimes take the train to Vicksburg and Jackson, Mississippi or Monroe, Louisiana. She called those trips "taking a joy." Even though her trip to Oakland would bring her to a new life with new struggles with old obligations of hard work, that trip was to Mildred very much like "taking a joy." "I liked that train ride. Passing by people waving. Look out and talk to different people riding with you. Make friends with the people at the station until, Choo-choo!" Soon though, the further west they traveled, the tougher the trip became. "Everywhere we

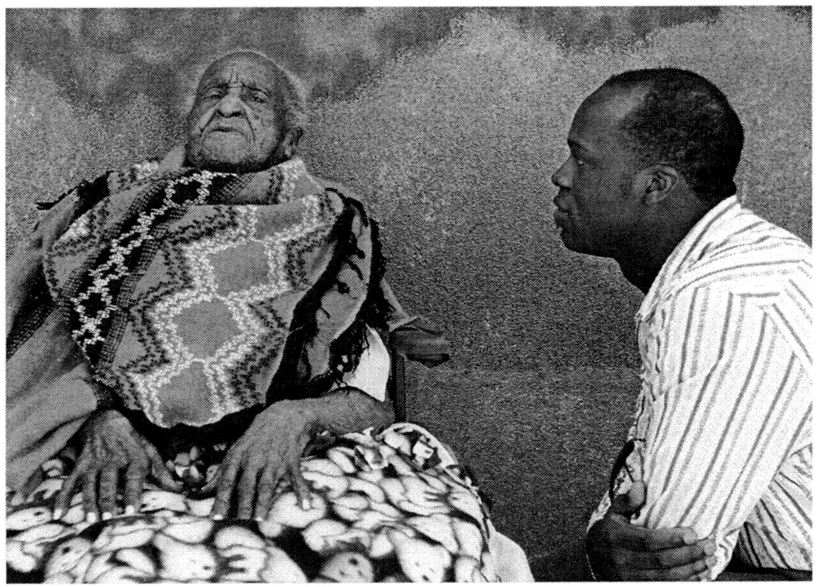

Mildred with her writer, Cleavon

stopped for food and water, they'd be fresh out, and the children, ohhh-we, they would get to crying." She shakes her head and looks away. Then looking back at me, crossing her wrists and pressing them against her chest, "I'm so glad Benny wasn't with me then. I would have grabbed him and jumpt out the window to see him crying so."

Immediately the trip ends...

When Mildred told me about this trip, it was two months into her work with me. In this time she had told me the names of the people in the photographs around her bed. She had computer-scanned print-outs of her grandfather and grandmother, George and Susan Knapper. There was one of her sister Etta's sons along with his family dressed in summer clothes and all smiles. There was a photograph of her mother and one of her father and one of Mildred, herself around the age of her parents in their photos. I knew a little about the people scotch-taped to the walls or door near her bed, and in time I had planned to ask more, but I had never heard of Benny, the son she would have jumped out of a moving train for to keep from having to hear his crying like those starving, thirsty children on her train ride out to Oakland.

Benny is her seventy-five-year-old son who is old enough to have retired recently from a second career, but to hear Mildred talk of him one would think he were still in grade school.

Benny is her seventy-five-year-old son who is old enough to have retired recently from a second career, but to hear Mildred talk of him one would think he were still in grade school. "He was the nicest boy. He absolutely was. Boys would fight; he wouldn't fight 'em back. My papa, he say, 'Mildred,' he says, 'you got one of the nicest kids.' And he had to be if my father say so." Mildred's arms, wrists, and fingers, her neck and tongue and eyes all twitch when she talks of Benny. It's not a nervous twitching, but rather the twitching like a child waiting for a long deserved treat or a mother longing to hold her babe.

"He was always in a rush." She rushes to tell me. She shakes her head in mock disapproval of his flinging himself from one task to another. "He'd come in saying, 'Mama, did you see?' and I'd say, 'Boy, don't run so.' Everywhere he had to run to." She holds the "ru" in "rush" and "run" in her throat and presses her diaphragm to emphasize his "rushing" and "running."

So much she tells me about Benny. Like a charmer of ropes and snakes, she charms my pen. It falls, and I listen. All I can do is listen. When I come to visit and Mildred is tired and depressed, we talk about Benny.

When I want to see Mildred smile, we talk about Benny. When I am tired and depressed and need to witness unconditional love, we talk about her little boy, Benny.

"Children had a price for going for something. It was a nickel, but Benny never asked for a nickel." Her pride can't be hidden, and it's hard to imagine how youth could add any more body English to the affection for her son she holds. Once when she's done telling me how they sang hymns together, she smacks her tongue against the roof of her mouth with the pace of a slow rocking chair. Mother and son singing together ("He would hum to my songs, and I would hum to his") the two singing together, rocking in time. "When Benny was off in the service, ohhhh. I felt like...ohhhh. That grieved me. It grieved me till I cried. All I could think about was how we used to sit in the chair and sing together."

Like a charmer of ropes and snakes, she charms my pen. It falls, and I listen.

Benny's grown and retired now. She tells me of his recent second retirement, the pride makes her body shiver. "He worked so hard. Yeah, from a little boy." She remembers a recent conversation the two had. He was telling her how much work he had done in his life. She humphs a smile. "Then he said, 'I'm not telling you what it took to get here because you already know.'"

Yes, Mildred knows. Again. Place and being. Here. Where she is, who she is. Here. One looking back on a life of work-service. Here. Oakland. She had committed herself to jumping out of a moving train with her son if he had cried so like the other thirsty, hungry children on that trip from Louisiana. But his birth was further down the line, and Mildred arrived in Oakland. "Came out here by myself. I got on the train, but I didn't know I was going that fur [sic]."

It was tough at first. "You couldn't get a garage to live in with so many people. Everybody any color. Everybody slept where they could. You were lucky if you could get somewhere with your work. The Mexicans worked all day and fell right out of there into their beds or people just piled up in a room." Mildred was one of the luckier ones, though. There was a couple from Louisiana who had a room. They got a better job, moved, and Mildred took their room in a Victorian in West Oakland off 15th Street with only a bed and dresser. She was lucky. "If you could get a room, you got a palace."

As she puts it, "I knew some people, had a place to live and went

Cannery or laundry jobs were the only ones African Americans emigrating from the South could get at the time, other than jobs working in the fields.

to work. [I] worked at the Del Monte cannery on East 14th Street canning peaches, pears, apples, tomatoes. All from Oakland." She adds the last sentence to remind me how much has changed, how long she's been here.

She worked machines for cutting fruit. "Nice shiny machines. I don't know whether [it's] because I ain't seen no machines, but it was so clean. Long belts and you could stand on each side and men dump fruit on the belt and people on each side would sort and take 'em out and grab all the fruit off the belt and put it in a can. I was the cutter. This is me." She starts miming working on the line by tapping with one fingertip the table that rolls alongside her bed and swivels over her chest so that she can have her dinners. Then, swooping with the opposite hand the spot where her finger had just tapped. She smiles and clicks her nails on the table, flipping the imaginary fruit over her shoulders. "Just that fast. The fruit on that machine." I can't imagine a twenty-year-old moving any faster. "I mean the whole eight hours we worked that way, and can you believe what we got paid? Sixty-five cents an hour. Now people makes more money sitting down. They pay eight or nine dollars and these people ain't doing a dime worth of work."

Cannery or laundry jobs were the only ones African Americans emigrating from the South could get at the time, other than jobs working in the fields. And field work was different from any Mildred had done in Louisiana, not because of the crop or the temperature but because, for the first time, she would work someone else's land.

One of her brothers who had been "running the road" had gotten California in her head. "No harm done in California; everything is blue skies," he had told her. "Who wouldn't wanna go somewhere where you'd be happy, where you could work and make some good, clean money? But to tell the truth, I didn't see no difference. You could press a button to get your water, but other than that it was worse in California than back home. While we chopped cotton, the guy standing in back of the wagon just telling you to work, and if you didn't, they had someone waiting to take your place." As she talks her jaws get full. She's mad. She grabs the rail by her head and pulls herself closer to me. "Never had nothing like that in Louisiana...I was running from the devil and ran right into his arms. It was the same. If you went somewhere where the white folks was, you had to go in the backdoor."

Oakland wouldn't ever live up to the image her brother had painted for the impressionable teen-ager before she moved out, but blue skies had never been anything Mildred needed for spirit. She continued to work. She went from the factories and the fields and on to the Oak Knoll Naval Hospital where she cared for the repatriated prisoners of war returning from the South Pacific. "When I worked up there, it wasn't nothing but eucalyptus trees, one gas station, and one church."

She took other jobs, and when the work she did for wages didn't provide more than a capitalistic service to a community beyond herself, she began working for the NAACP making lunch for picketers and joining them as they worked/served for more job opportunities for African Americans in Oakland.

"People used to be good people, but it went away somewhere, and I just don't understand."

Thinking about her work in those days reminds me of what she said once about what she had learned from working on her family farm. She told me, "When [my brothers, sister and I] got on our own, we kept doing. It was hard back then, but when you looked around, you could see some joy in doing it." The joy for Mildred was helping others.

"People used to be good people, but it went away somewhere, and I just don't understand." Later she tells me, "People just don't have no heart no more. What done happened...what done happened...I don't know. She hits a blue note when she finished the sentence, the last syllable is hardly audible, for her throat strains the breath needed for her words; she's making the softest most important note a singer could produce.

She had always helped others. She helped Tillman Williams, an usher at Mt. Zion on 12th and Waller. She helped a woman named Olivia Allen on Friday through Sunday nights, leaving on Monday morning until Ms. Allen had a stroke. Mildred had put shoes on her, fixed her some meat and set it out on the table. Mildred did the cleaning and the cooking of the meals. She helped both of these people traveling from one end of Oakland to the other riding a bus.

Now she finds herself at the point where she most needs the help of others, which is where I find her, crying from pain and neglect, from love, *for* love. I'm at her door and she's obviously in pain. I tiptoe in because I'm not sure she's awake. The curtains of the window to her left are closed. When she hears me, she's startled not knowing who I am. I greet her good afternoon to give her a chance to remember me. Before recognition flashes

I stay with Mildred because I am too afraid of what my wanting to leave reveals about me.

in her eyes, I can see the pain she's in. There is no separation of the physical from the emotional or the spiritual for Mildred. When she is in pain, her whole being aches, and I know it. She calls on the Lord to understand her pain and how it makes it hard to be faithful. "Mister" she calls to me shaking her head. This is early in our relationship. I am still uncomfortable going to Willow Tree. I am still uncomfortable with the smell that I have, in my ignorance, equated with death. I am forced to realize that I had hoped Mildred would give me a chance to feel good today. I have come wanting her to tell me some story that would make both of us smile so that I could go home and rejoice in life without having to regard it in its entirety. I feel that I am already upset with Mildred for being in pain. I want to leave, but I stay. Not because I have been pulled by the power of the longing in her eyes, not because I want to console Mildred, not because I want to use Mildred as a medium through which I could feel that I were consoling the universe. I stay with Mildred because I am too afraid of what my wanting to leave reveals about me.

She begins to complain that some people just don't help her out. Then she tells me, "Ever since I was big enough to carry a bucket across a field I been trained to help people. It stayed in me until these old feet put me down." I am made to realize that work and helping people are linked in Mildred's eyes, her sense of being. She can no longer work or help people. And what she wants so badly, she feels is not reciprocated. Why after all of her helping people from such an early age is she not being helped as she deserved?

"I'd rather be under the bridge than in here." She tells me, her words floating through the air like puffs of smoke through her trembling lips. "Now is the worse time I've ever had. I can't get off my back. So sore sometimes I cry through the night." Her face is crying. It is a clear day, so I go over to open the curtains to the window. She begins to sing, "Stay with me, Jesus. Jesus, please stay with me. I know you with me, and as long as you with me I know I'm not alone. Stay with me, Jesus."

A bird bounces in the evergreen shrub outside her window. I ask her if she can see it. We begin to talk about birds. "Good stuff God put on for us here to enjoy. Birds and bees...that's life. It's terrible..." Her eyes show a different kind of pain. "It's a shame how we ain't got so many of these birds now. Deprived of God's gifts. It's music to your heart. I don't care when they come, they welcome to my sight and my ear."

She begins to tell me about a farm in Louisiana. The farm is the home of the woman lying in the bed before me. She tells me about work and service. She tells me she had lots of cousins and friends, but lots of work to do and no time to play. She tells me about playing and walking a friend home back and forth both unable to say good-bye. She tells me about a train ride to California when she defiantly rode in a seat next to a white woman. The woman in the bed before me is that woman staring the white woman down. She tells me about playing checkers with Ms Pecola Berry every night, and about getting peanuts at the Swan Market in downtown Oakland. She tells me how her landlord, Ms Esteeve would give her a ride to work if she were ever late. She laughs and says "Me and Benny's first wife used to do some of the stupidest things."

She's working on me, teaching me who she is. She's doing her service for me, making me capable of seeing a person for the life she has lived rather than for the tears she cries.

She's doing her service for me, making me capable of seeing a person for the life she has lived rather than for the tears she cries.

I originally thought Mildred was my project, but in time I saw how I was actually hers. Instead of finding the details of her life and molding them into a story, her story molded me into a person capable of seeing her life not as a listing of facts or a narrative arc. She also taught me to see beyond the tears in her eyes to go beyond them to understand that the moments of her crying, the moments of her fears of dying, her frustration of ending her life in a nursing home are only those: moments. And those moments when calculated with the other moments of her life create a beautiful mosaic to honor and respect and celebrate.

Later she will tell me, "All the bad things have come down on me, but you share with me the good. The good is what we say to one another to pick us up and give us something to go home laughing with." She calls and I respond.

I say, "But the good things are more than that. Through these good things we find faith."

"Yes," she calls back. "Faith is the right word. Through faith, good will prevail."

And goodness lies in this bed, in this room, in this city far from Tallulah, Louisiana. I can see it now. And I can see strength. In this body, in this being that months ago I would have called weak. And I believe their words now, those who say it is for the strong to protect the weak.

But to accept their words we have to see how our idea of strength is skewed. When I first met Mildred lying in her bed, her body covered by a faded robe and almost melted into the mattress of the bed, I hardly appreciated or respected her. I saw her as weak. I saw myself as someone who would "make" her into a person we should respect and value, ignorant of the fact that each day I would see her, her strength would overshadow me like an autumn evening cloud slowly dimming the lights of the moon. With each lesson, yes, now I am coming to realize that Mildred didn't share with me stories, she shared lessons, and with each lesson, Mildred taught me a truer idea of strength. Any measure of strength by any means other than love and compassion is not a measure of strength all. Mildred is strong and with her love of life and community of work and service she can protect us. With only two teeth, without being able to leave her bed, she has tried to protect me from a less than natural way of seeing the world. ■

When I first met Mildred lying in her bed, her body covered by a faded robe and almost melted into the mattress of the bed, I hardly appreciated or respected her.

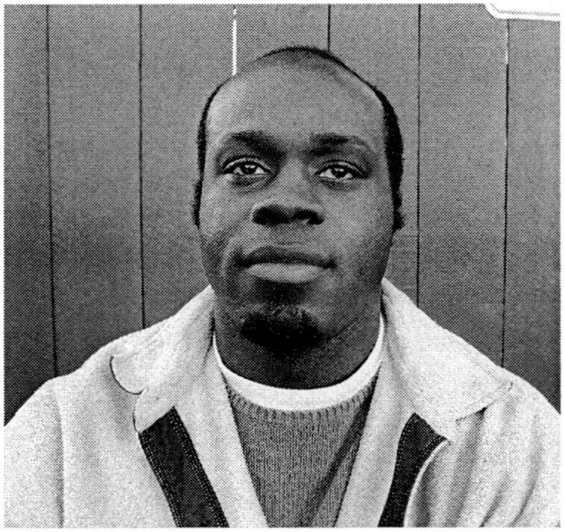

Cleavon Smith

I have an MFA in English and Creative Writing from Mills College, and currently teach at Vista Community College and Patten University. On a volunteer basis, I work with youth, grades K-12, teaching poetry and creative writing as well as facilitating bereavement groups.

At the beginning of this project, I wanted to learn a little about aging and my reactions to it, but I also wanted to reconnect with the South. Not just the kudzu and the humidity —the South is nothing without it's people—I wanted to reconnect with the spirit, the strength, the sense of humor, and the will of the South, that place where I lived from birth until the day I left to go to the Naval Academy at seventeen.

Working with Mildred I received all that I had wanted and much, much more. Usually I spend my time writing stories and beginning novels with characters I've created to deal with issues I've chosen to face, but with Mildred I learned how the soul determines, if not all, a great deal of our being—how we choose to influence and react to the world. She also helped me to understand the variety of stories, the amazing complexities, and the magnitude of dreams burning inside the people living in nursing facilities throughout the country. Mildred brought me closer to my own family, by sharing with me her story and her relationship with her family. By showing me how she is connected both to Oakland and her hometown, she also brought me closer to being able to call both Oakland and Baldwyn, Mississippi my home.

The *Nine Lives* project isn't just connecting the generations; it's educating and celebrating lives!

VIRGINIA HOLLAND

Lawton Health Care Center
San Francisco, California
with
Victoria S. Cormack

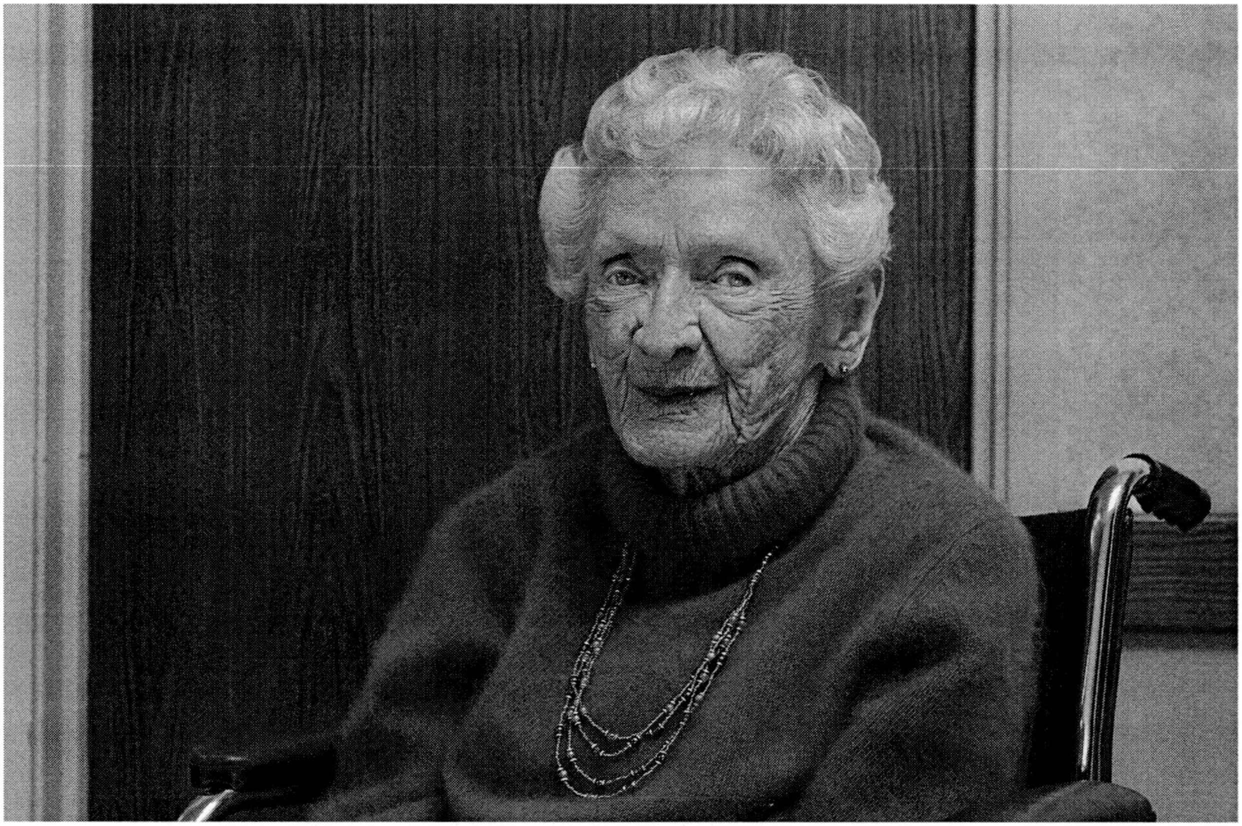

"Life has been good to me"

Virginia Holland sits at the end of a long corridor, her face illuminated by the skylights at Lawton Health Care Center in San Francisco. She's dressed in the colors of the flowers that surround the long-term care facility and blossom in the community garden across the street. She looks as though she should either be lovingly tending the garden or giving a tour. Virginia, whom I'll come to know as "Gini," awaits me like an anticipatory bride or mother waiting to birth her story. From her wheelchair, she waves as I approach and her face lights up when I bend closely to her ear so she can hear me ask, "And how are you doing today?"

Meeting a person for the first time is always an uncertain adventure, but somehow this seems like a grander event. Gini has agreed to tell me her story, and I want to share it with all the dignity with which she offers it. But my trepidation proves unnecessary as Gini falls easily into conversation, pulling out a photo of her newest great-grandchild, Karenna Inez. The baby's head is covered with a big shock of black hair and her gorgeous, round, brown eyes stare directly at her father.

Hers is the tale of raising a family in Southern California over five decades, of nurturing an ever-widening circle of family—which now includes grandchildren and great-grandchildren.

Over the weeks, I come to understand the multilayered dimensions of interrelationships, names and current places of residence of Gini's family. In the storytelling, these people will become living emblems sewn onto the sleeve of Gini's life and purpose. Hers is the tale of raising a family in Southern California over five decades, of nurturing an ever-widening circle of family—which now includes grandchildren and great-grandchildren.

Like many women of her generation, Virginia centered her life on the abundant tasks and joys of raising a family. I grew up with my older brother and my mother, a single working parent, who sometimes held down more than one job to support us. Now I myself am raising a son and three cats as a single parent, while finishing my graduate degree and working as a journalist and gerontologist. I also act as the primary caregiver for my mother, who resides in an independent living facility and always claims to be slightly older than the comedian Jack Benny, who was eternally thirty-nine. Although mine is a small biological family, our lives are rich, with the extended family full of beloved friends, some old and some very new.

The world Virginia describes is like something out of a novel or an old television series, but it does not parallel my upbringing. Hers is the story of the family next door to Ozzie and Harriet. But there is a sense of struggle in her story that none of the Nelson's let on about. The "ideal" Nelson family or even that of the Cleavers (remember the Beaver's mom?), portrayed in popular '50s TV programs, never moved. Harriet, unlike Gini, didn't have to deal with the challenge of setting up new homes and enrolling her children in different schools to accompany Ozzie's frequent transfers during World War II. There was never divorce, dissent or illness, but that was TV. Still Gini, not unlike Harriet, asserts, "I have no regrets; life has been good to me."

Gini talks about her children during every visit, turning over the stories like a gem with infinite facets and holding it up to the brilliant light of day. She has three children—Steven, George and Raymond. Though she may forget the specifics of a story or which son did what, her voice is always full of pride and love. "I live on memories, that's all that is left," she admits, with tears in her luminous blue eyes. I pass her a tissue, comfort her, and after a deep breath, she continues on with her story.

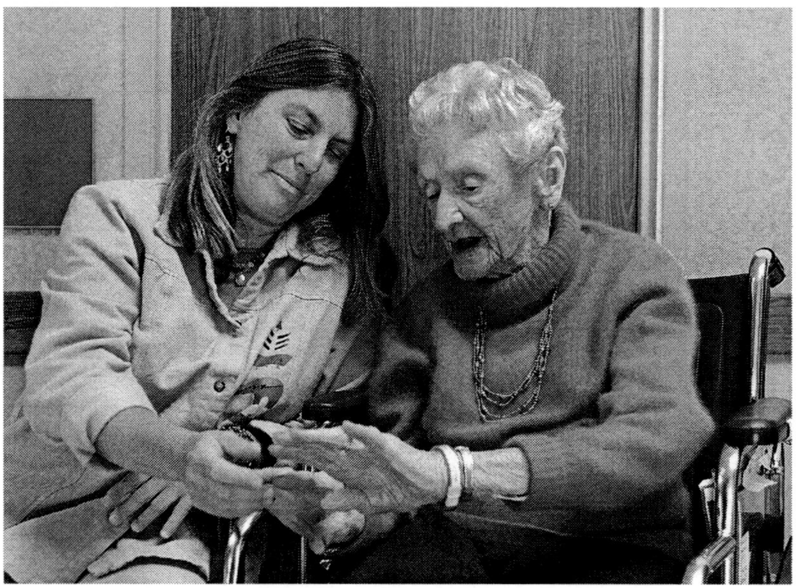

Virginia and her writer, Victoria

Today Gini lives with the realization that she is the last one standing in a room that used to be filled with life, family and friends—the last of her generation, of her peer group. "My mother and father were in their eighties [when they passed away]. They weren't as old as I am now," she says. Her younger sister Jean, the only other child of their parents George Rowe and Marie Franz, is gone now also. She was born three years later and was, as Gini lovingly describes her, "the size of an Easter basket."

Gini cherishes a remarkable collection of exquisite photos of her ancestors. Gini's maternal grandfather, the youngest of eighteen children, came to the U.S. from Germany, married Gini's grandmother, Mary

Franz, who already had four children. The marriage didn't last long—Ludvig, a wealthy "gay young blade," as Gini describes him, wasn't a good match for Mary Franz, a practical, self-sufficient woman who worked as a nurse. Gini's mother, Marie, was young when they divorced, but Gini still remembers her Grandpa Ludvig with obvious affection. "He could not do enough for us and bought us all we wanted. We had gold watches before any of the other children!" On Sundays, he'd take her sister and her to the zoo. "It was fun to go to parks back in the '20s, when the streetcars substituted for automobiles, " she adds.

For a while, Harvey was "interested in older girls," Gini says coyly, explaining that he was two years older than she was.

Later Gini's grandmother took on a job caring for a wealthy family and became known in the neighborhood as "Auntie Franz." Gini was proud to be a direct descendant of the famous "Auntie Franz," who came to achieve almost movie star status in the Des Moines neighborhood.

Gini's mother, Marie, grew up in Des Moines and worked as a teacher in the Des Moines schools. Her father, George Rowe, was a banker until the Great Depression, which Gini refers to as "the failure." Her memories of her childhood are spotty until she becomes a young woman and wife of Harvison (Harvey) Holland.

Gini's and Harvey's was a storybook romance. Their families had lived only blocks away in the same Des Moines neighborhood. For a while, Harvey was "interested in older girls," Gini says coyly, explaining that he was two years older than she was. And like Gini's grandparents, Harvey's parents were divorced. Gini comments, "I think I knew Harvey's dad better than he did," since Harvey's father lived on the same streetcar line as Gini.

Gini studied for a double major, in dietetics and institutional management at Iowa State University. Her social life centered on her sorority and she wrote for the society section of the school newspaper. She also worked part-time at an insurance office. But her education—and her student life—were radically altered by a sudden change in wedding plans.

As a specialist in aeronautical engineering, educated at Annapolis and Iowa State, Harvey received a call in March of 1934 offering him a permanent position in Northern California. The catch was that he had to appear the next day for work.

"I already had my engagement ring," Gini explains, "but we did not have a date set for the wedding; we thought about June." The couple jumped at the chance of moving across the country—no more cold weather and a permanent home. Gini's mom and Harvey spent all day getting a special license and arranged for the wedding that evening. They then immediately got on the plane to California. "I only had five quarters of PE left," she admits, with no tone of regret in her voice. Instead, she laughs and continues, "That sounds a lot like a soap opera, doesn't it?" She was twenty at the time.

Among many people of my generation, in an age when the term "family" is being redefined in a myriad of ways, the decision to sacrifice work or education for family life would be a difficult one. Gini seemed to be ahead of the curve; there was no doubt, nor real choice, for Gini and Harvey but to follow the opportunity.

Gini now describes herself as a "sturdy old woman," but it's obvious to me that she has been "sturdy" throughout her life, adapting readily to new places. Once in California, there was a lot of moving in the first few years. They spent only a year in Burlingame, when Harvey worked at the San Francisco Airport, before the family relocated. When their first son George was two, they were transferred to a town outside Dayton, Ohio, headquarters of the Air Force. They lived in a temporary residence for families who worked in the airplane industry. War was threatening and as a designer and airplane engineer, his skills were in great demand.

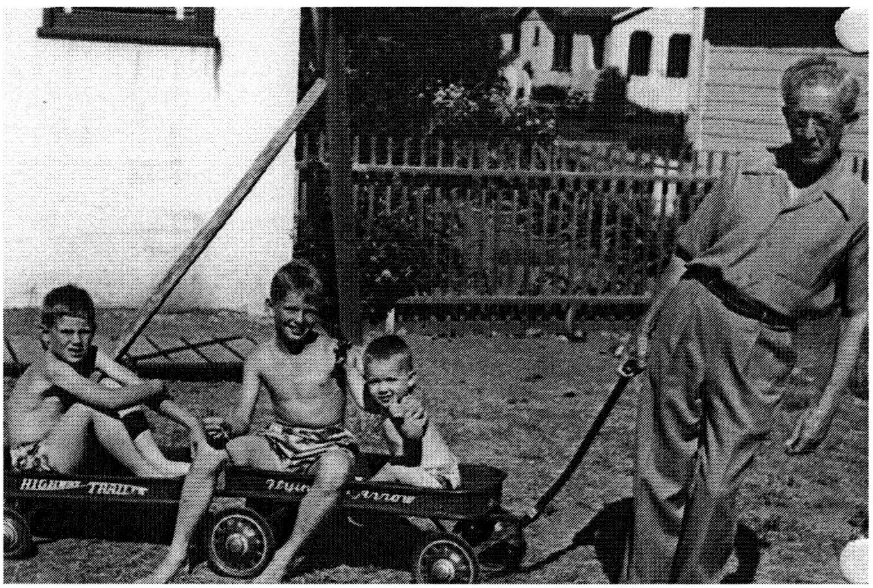

Harvey takes his sons for a ride

When she reflects on the family's frequent moves, Gini says, "We had no choice. If you wanted a good job and fair pay, you went." Revealing her remarkable ability to see the bright side of life, she also sees the benefits for her sons:

"It was the best thing that could have happened to my boys. It helped them learn how to make friends and adapt to new situations."

Even at three months of age, the Holland's son George was getting a lesson in adapting. Gini recalls taking him on an early airplane flight that she took to Des Moines to help celebrate her parents' twenty-fifth wedding anniversary. "There were no planes for civilians," she explains. Since she didn't know when the flight arrived, she says, "I just called when I got there. I got a free pass, but there were no seat belts, so you had to hang on!"

The kids got along well she recalls, but they had their share of "requisite disagreements."

Through the many moves, Gini seems to keep track of the years by remembering the emergencies and early childhood traumas of her sons. George broke his collarbone, and Ray his leg in those early years. When neighbors saw Gini carrying Ray, who was a "big boy," home from the doctor's office, they would offer her their porch stoop as a place for the two to rest.

The Holland's youngest son, Steven, was born near the end of the war. The kids got along well, she recalls, but they had their share of "requisite disagreements." Gini offers with a gentle laugh: "Each one had his own mind." She emphasizes that the "older ones took care of the little ones." Gini recalls an incident when Raymond stood up and demanded, "Mom, say something to me, just to Ray." Gini admits she "felt terrible" when she recognized in his plea that it wasn't easy being the middle son. Ray, she adds, attended five schools in the first years of his life.

Steven, too, had his share of childhood traumas. He was hit by a car when he was small and lost a kidney. Because his physical condition precluded his participation in the contact sports that his brothers enjoyed, he became a wonderful swimmer. His talents even earned him "adoption" by a local swim club.

When Gini was a young mother, she liked to take the boys on road trips. One of her road trip memories clearly reveals the efforts she'd make to maintain the family connections. She and her sister Jean (who lived in Lincoln, Nebraska)—with their families in tow— rendezvoused in a town midway between their two homes. The challenge was finding a place to stay with such a big crowd, which included many children. "We packed up our car [and headed] for Hannibal, Missouri. It was just a great place between Lincoln and Dayton. They had big rooms and a couple of cribs. There was room for everyone."

In the '40s, the Holland family moved to Southern California, near the West Los Angeles area where I grew up in the late '50s and through the '60s. I've been back only a few times after the death of my grandmother Beatrice Bachmann in the late '80s. It was she who played a vital role in my upbringing and introduced me to her world—of wise older people with exceptional stories—and to her exuberant but slower life. And so it was with special interest that I listened to this part of Gini's story, though our stories were very different.

"I didn't want to be cut off from everything, and it [volunteer work] was one way to keep in touch."

I was raised in an apartment south of Wilshire Boulevard in Beverly Hills, the daughter of a secretary working in the fast-paced film industry. The Holland's odyssey in Los Angeles is that of a dream realized, of coming of age in a town as it was blooming and offering possibilities to new families who flooded in from the Midwest and East Coast. These people might have been my neighbors. Gini could have been one of the women I passed in the stores on Beverly Drive or on my many walks to Santa Monica beach in my teens. Perhaps it was her driving her passel of children to sports, soccer, baseball and swimming, while I browsed bookstores in Westwood or the shops on Sunset Boulevard. We compare notes on the feeling of exhaustion after day trips to Disneyland and Knott's Berry Farm. While Gini and Harvey took their youngest son, Steven, to the well-known amusement parks, family and friends shared the experience with me, since my mother did not drive.

Gini is still proud of the "big house" she kept, "four bedroom, two stories in Santa Monica, off San Vicente [Blvd.]." They moved there, originally, she says, because they couldn't afford Beverly Hills and they wanted a good school system for the boys. Gini stayed at home until the youngest son, Steven, was five.

With the boys enrolled in school during the daytime, she then began volunteer work, extending her circle of caring beyond the reach of her own family. "I did work, anything I could get," she asserts. "I didn't want to be cut off from everything, and it [volunteer work] was one way to keep in touch." She was the "birthday lady" at a school for children with cerebral palsy. Her job was to bring a big sheet cake, which she decorated for all the celebrations at the center. She still remembers how all the children would clap when they saw her. "I took my boys so that they would know about volunteers and helping others," she says. Gini also worked in a type of adoption agency, which placed babies with families. Gini went beyond her role as head of the household to expand her concept of community to include those in her town, neighborhood and work. I am again impressed by her generosity of spirit and her belief in extending the circle of family.

The family also expanded, at one time, to include Harvey's mother, who came to live with the family in her elder years. She drove a car until she reached her seventies and Gini laughs remembering the family's six cars, so abundant that Harvey had to create assigned parking spaces behind the house.

Gini is a self-described "wizard" in the kitchen. She was good at picking, freezing and cooking, aided by her education as a dietician. *The Joy of Cooking* is her favorite cookbook, and of course she used to watch "the lady from TV, with her own show, Julia Child." She talks about all the entertaining she did, preparing and serving food on china for thirty-five or forty neighbors. "We also had community potlucks and everyone brought something different," she recalls. She even taught the boys to cook, a skill she has tried to pass on to her grandchildren as well. She was very involved, too, in church-related functions at the Westwood Hills Christian Church, where Harvey was a deacon for many years.

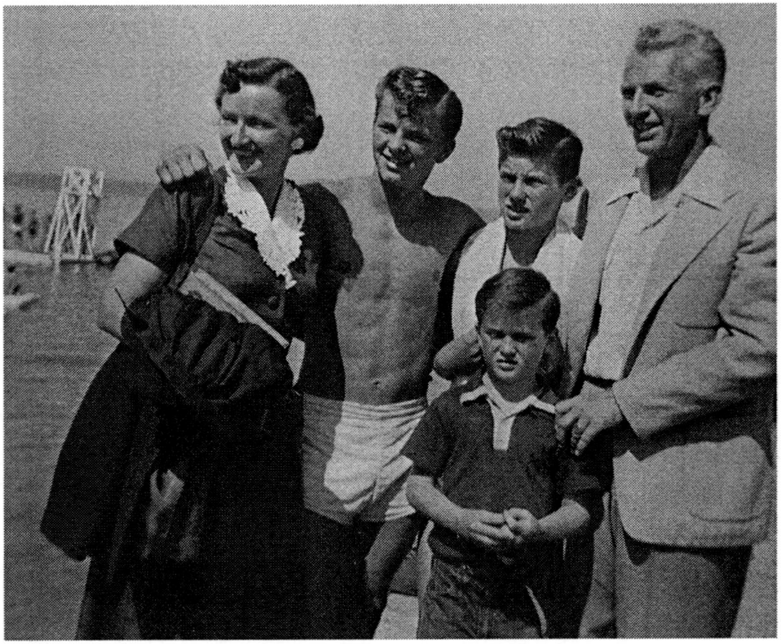

The Holland family on Catalina Island

During our conversations, Gini shares with me a comical "bad hair tale." She used to get her hair done at Bullock's Westwood, a fashionable department store in the Westwood district of Los Angeles. It was a place where my own mother and grandmother used to dress up and go for tea and finger sandwiches. One day her regular hairdresser was out and his substitute dyed her hair an "awful orange." She had a doctor's appointment immediately afterwards, and she still remembers how the people in the doctor's office "just cringed when they saw my hair." She returned immediately afterwards to the beauty salon for a color change.

Even after their departure, her sons continue to be essential to her sense of self, well-being, joy and peace of mind.

Once in their Santa Monica house, the Holland family continued their numerous excursions. "When we could afford it, we traveled to many places; we spent a lot of time in Mexico where it was cheap and safe." Though they didn't speak Spanish, they "went most anyplace," Gini recalls of their frequent trips there. With the Mexican border so close to Los Angeles, they went whenever they could. One of my favorite photos in her collection is a 1950s black-and-white image with the Holland family car in the foreground, on an unpaved street lined with booths selling Mexican crafts.

With three sons, Harvey delighted in taking them hunting and fishing. Harvey had been raised using guns in the Midwest, and often took the boys on his trips. Gini still remembers the pheasants they brought home. "They are wonderful eating; the boys dressed and froze them. Eventually we had to get a freezer cabinet until we ate them."

Fishing, too, provided memories of plentiful harvests. After a successful fishing excursion to Mexico, Harvey, the boys and some friends came home with twenty-seven albacore—so many that they had to become "professional" fish packers on the spot. "We could hardly get it into the freezer, and set up a packaging area in the back yard!" Gini smiles mischievously when she explains that the Hollands took the prime cuts for themselves. Harvey halved them and the boys trimmed, while she did the packaging. After first distributing what they could to the neighbors, they went down to the pier and sold the rest commercially.

But the boys who used to spend time with dad on fishing and hunting expeditions eventually grew into adulthood to leave the family "nest." Even after their departure, her sons continue to be essential to her sense of self, well-being, joy and peace of mind. All attended college and graduated with honors, a point of great pride for Gini. George and Ray went to UCLA; Steven received a Ph.D. in forestry from University of California at Santa Barbara. In total, her sons have blessed her with five grandchildren, ages five to forty, and three great - grandchildren, ages eight, twelve, and sixteen.

Their stories are like those of their generation, with their share of joys and heartbreaks, marriages and divorces—Gini tells about them as if they were her own, and they are.

Steven married during his student years at University of California at Santa Barbara, and his daughter Lisa arrived early in their marriage, shortly after his wife graduated from high school. "Steve's wife was darling about working," explains Gini. "We did not subsidize them." They rented a home in the hills of Santa Barbara overlooking the university. One of Gini's favorite stories involves a very little girl and a very big dog. With her mother working, and her father completing his degree, Lisa was left to go to school herself. They found a pedigreed Dalmatian at the pound to accompany the youngster on the long walk to the bus stop, where she picked up her bus to school. The dog watched over her granddaughter, giving Gini some piece of mind. Knowing the importance of family to Gini, I can imagine her worry and concern about Lisa.

When the marriage ended, Steve tried to find a job with his newly acquired degree. He eventually became a trail guide and forest ranger, working in Alaska, at Yellowstone and Yosemite. Steve makes his present home in the Tetons, surrounding himself with nature and getting together with family during his yearly visits.

It was his daughter Lisa who dubbed Gini with her family nickname, "Ginigrams." But even though Lisa is now a mother herself, Gini continues to worry about her. The little girl who once walked to the bus stop with her big Dalmatian now works at Nipomo Prison and her job requires that she carry a gun. "Ginigrams, don't worry about it," Lisa admonishes her grandmother about the possibility of having to use the weapon. But worry is one thing that is hard for the matriarch of the family to let go of.

Gini helped raise the twin daughters of her oldest son, George, who divorced when he was younger and now lives with his new wife in Chicago. After his divorce, his ex-wife moved to India, leaving George with the responsibility of raising Kira and Krista. George retired early from his job as an English professor and brought the girls to L.A. to be near their grandparents. "It nearly broke my heart," she admits, when the time came to send the girls to visit their mother in an ashram—an experience quite distant from her own upbringing in Des Moines. But Gini dutifully dressed the twins in matching shirts and plaid skirts and jackets and put them on the plane to India. Her concern ended only when the girls returned safely. Her comment brings back memories of my own spontaneous road trips and the worry I must have caused my family when I would call unexpectedly from Yosemite one day and then Boulder a few days later.

Ray, who lives in San Francisco and is Gini's primary caregiver, worked as an attorney after graduating from UCLA. Gini beams when she tells how "right after the wedding, they [Ray and his wife Melinda] went into the Peace Corps in Venezuela and lived there for two years in the '60s." It is quite an exotic story for a boy who grew up in Los Angeles, yet it fits with the underlying theme in the Holland family story, of traveling and adapting to new places. Still, I can imagine Gini worrying when any bit of disquieting news from Latin America appeared on TV or in the newspaper. It was Ray and Melinda who hosted Gini's 90th birthday party. All the children pitched in to have a party and practically everyone in the family managed to attend the special occasion. It's one of Gini's fondest memories in this, her later life.

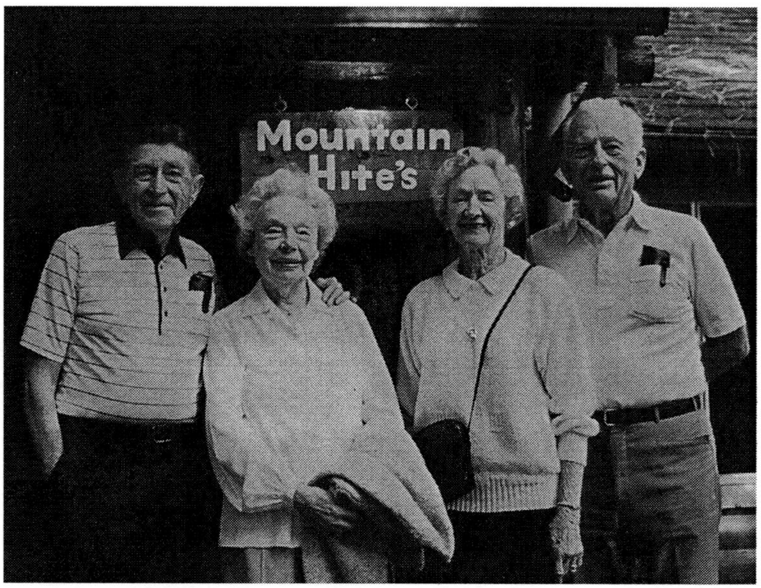

Virginia and Harvey (at right) with their friends Felicia and Dick Crane on vacation at Wawona, 1991

Gini's ninetieth birthday had been preceded by a much sadder occasion, which also drew the family together—the funeral of Gini's husband Harvey. For many years, the couple had enjoyed living the life of "empty nesters" as their sons established their own paths. Symbolic of that time is a photo near Gini's bed in her room at Lawton. It's of Harvey and Gini in front of the Eiffel Tower. The Hollands traveled extensively, often with their dearest friends Dick and Felicia Crane, taking cruises and enjoying their favorite sports of golf and swimming wherever they could.

Harvey "couldn't sit still" after his retirement at the age of sixty-five, says Gini. "He was a "darned good mechanic," and immediately set to restoring to perfect condition an original chocolate brown Mustang. Harvey turned his backyard into an urban farm, growing everything from fruits (even blueberries from Georgia) and vegetables to flowers. According to Gini, they didn't buy any fresh produce for twenty years, and graciously shared their "crops" with their neighbors. She describes an idyllic Los Angeles scene, of people stopping in the alley and talking over the back fence to Harvey in his backyard—it was a part of Los Angeles I never saw growing up.

"It's what's left over once the butcher has cut it, mixed with corn meal and spices. It's everything but the squeal!"

The Hollands celebrated their marriage by renewing their vows at their twenty-fifth and fiftieth anniversaries. To me, the symbolism of this gesture spoke to the strength of their union over the decades. It seemed only fitting then, that the minister who married them, a cousin in the family, also presided over Harvey's funeral service, which was attended by the family and the Cranes.

After Harvey died in his eighties, Gini moved out of her house in Santa Monica to an apartment in an assisted living facility by the ocean. Gini gets wistful when she thinks of how the daughter of the famous folksinger Bob Dylan bought their family home, remodeling it in a way that changed it forever. "I couldn't bear to go in it now," she admits. With Gini's health challenges—vision problems and a fall that landed her in a wheelchair—her son Ray moved her to San Francisco where he could better monitor her care. It is he and his wife Melinda who launder her clothes and make weekly visits.

She admits that one of the greatest frustrations of aging is not being able to get up and go. On holidays like Easter, Gini still manages to get to Ray's house. "He has to carry me up the front stairs," she admits, but it's well worth the hassles to enjoy family again at her son's home over brunch. "We have scrapple. Do you know what that is?" she asks. I admit that I'm not familiar with the pork-based mush, which is shaped into loaves and then sliced for frying. "It's what's left over once the butcher has cut it, mixed with corn meal and spices. It's everything but the squeal!" On special occasions, like Mother's Day, Ray gets her out to local restaurants too.

She still loves to talk about food and sharing visits. When family isn't present, she depends on the images that surround her in her room. One of the photos in a prime viewing spot is that of Brook, the son of Ray and Melinda who is an attorney in New York, and his new daughter. She's happy

After looking back at her life, she concludes, "I have nothing to complain about."

that the family will be moving closer, to Spokane, and secretly hopes to see the baby more. Of Miles, Ray and Melinda's other son, she says proudly, "He is so good with older people, so kind and gentle." Miles, who works at Stanford, hopes to be a nurse practitioner. And she still keeps in touch with Dick Crane, who with his wife had been a frequent traveling companion of the Hollands. Like Gini, he too has lost his lifetime mate. "He's 98 and "deaf as a door," she confides with a giggle.

Even at ninety-one, Gini maintains a near-perfect appearance. Every time we meet, she has on a jewel-toned sweater and a beaded necklace. Her nails are beautifully manicured and she is dressed like she is ready for an outing. One of the aides at Lawton says she is always the first on Saturdays to get her hair done. "I don't like to wait," Gini explains. It seems to add to her sense of well-being. Her shiny exterior matches perfectly her positive outlook on life.

Gini celebrates graciously all that composes her life. She is full of sparkle, with a zest for bringing life to her abundant memories. She had devoted her life to making "room for everyone"—children, grandchildren, great-grandchildren, relatives and friends. She has made room for them all, nurturing her extended family with food and get-togethers, while she traveled the world by land, sea and air with a gypsy heart. After looking back at her life, she concludes, "I have nothing to complain about."

Our conversations about life in Southern California have reminded me of many aspects of my own childhood that I had forgotten to look at as I approach fifty and older adulthood. As a mother of another generation, I have come to admire Gini as a wise and caring mother and to appreciate the life she has led. Her story of kindness and generosity of spirit is one we can all learn from. ■

WRITER'S PROFILE

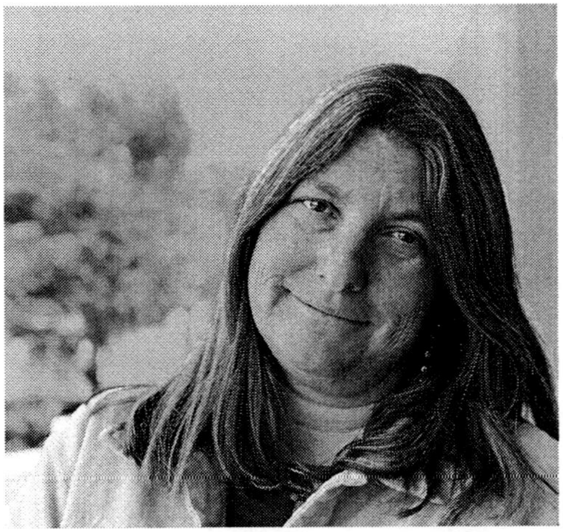

Victoria S. Cormack

I was born in Hungary and came to the U.S. at the age of two. Paradox is a big part of my vocabulary and life story. I grew up in West Los Angeles, where I and my brother John were raised by my mother and my grandmother. It was in Southern California where I gained an interest in social justice, writing, and community development.

As soon as I could, I transplanted myself to Northern California, where I've developed a rich circle of friends. I graduated from the University of California in Santa Cruz with a BA in community studies with an emphasis on Latin American Studies and an underlying interest in criminal justice and prisoners' rights. After working as a law librarian, paralegal and private investigator for nearly twenty years, I returned to school at San Francisco State, where I recently received an MA in gerontology, with an emphasis in journalism.

I am naturally nosy and love to write. As a freelance writer, I focus on developing resources for seniors and their caregivers, writing about stories of the disenfranchised and those without access to light and listeners. I have worked as a publications assistant, prison liaison, child advocate, second career instructor for seniors, and as a geriatric care coordinator.

During my long history of working with elders, I have accompanied them on appointments and sorted through the bureaucratic red tape of today's health care system. I have developed resources to help them remain at home and spoken up when their rights are denied. I currently am developing life review groups with elders. Writing Virginia Holland's life story has given me the opportunity to do something I love.

I also take care of my mother who lives in San Francisco, my ten-year-old son and three cats.

CHIZU IWATA

Mountain View Healthcare Center
Mountain View, California

with

Margaret S.A. Bacon

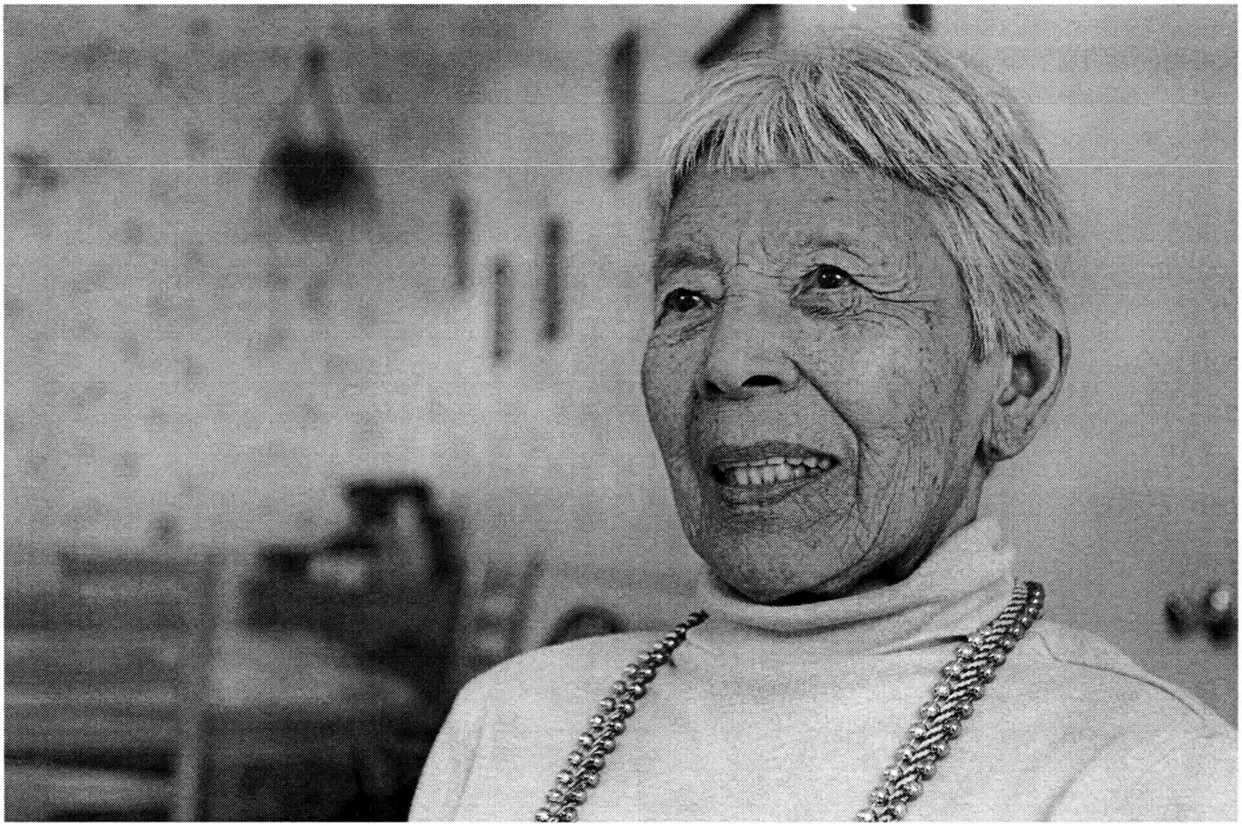

"I turned to flowers"

Every meeting with Chizu is a first. I always introduce myself and remind her that I am writing her story. Her brow furrows as she tries to remember me. She smiles and tells me that she vaguely recalls meeting me, but I know she is being polite. Still, she is always cheerful and friendly, sharing her stories willingly even though they are often the same stories she's told me before. I listen patiently and gently coax her to tell me more, knowing that eventually she'll share a tidbit of her life that is new to me. She easily slips back in time as if she is living at her home on Wright Avenue instead of the Mountain View Healthcare Center, working in her family's nursery, and driving her friends to *ikebana* meetings in San Francisco. Through Chizu I've come to appreciate the nebulous states of the past, present and future that we all drift in and out of.

Chizu was assigned to the Alzheimer's unit of Mountain View Healthcare Center shortly after Chizu and her brother, as her guardian, agreed to participate in the *Nine Lives* project. Still, it isn't until well into the project that I realize how advanced Chizu's memory loss really is. I have been visiting her every week for two months when I overhear another woman ask Chizu who I am.

"I don't know," Chizu tells her. "I've never seen her before in my life." Instead of being hurt, I am amused. For even though she may not remember me, I enjoy our visits. I believe Chizu does too.

We seem to connect on almost every visit, even if in her mind, we are becoming acquainted for the first time. I've come to realize that I can make a best friend for a day.

At our first meeting, Chizu smiles warmly and shakes my hand. I notice that her manicured nails are painted a metallic orange. A young color, I think. And as I come to know her, I realize she is young. She is animated and has a wonderful sense of humor. Chizu is a pretty woman, delicate and well-mannered, yet she has spunk. Her eyes flash and she laughs easily when she tells her tales.

Even though Chizu's short-term memory loss has made it difficult at times to piece together her story, I never wanted to abandon the project. We seem to connect on almost every visit, even if in her mind, we are becoming acquainted for the first time. I've come to realize that I can make a best friend for a day. On the bus, in a store, at the gym, I'll develop a wonderful rapport with someone only to never to see them again. Sort of like a platonic "one night stand." Perhaps Chizu is the same way. I've seen her chat cheerfully with other residents, banter with the health center staff and even flirt with a deliveryman with genuine affection. If she doesn't remember these people, then she is, indeed, meeting them for the first time.

And yet Chizu is aware of her poor memory. More than once she tells me, "I don't remember. You know, I'm a little bit this way," making circles with her finger at the side of her head. "Gee, it's pitiful to grow old," she adds wistfully.

Her brother, Roy, has told me that Chizu sometimes doesn't even recognize her own sisters. I've wondered if her friendliness is a way of compensating for her poor memory, so as not to offend someone when she doesn't remember them. And yet, I believe she is naturally gregarious and vivacious.

At our first meeting, she modestly says that she hasn't lived a very interesting life and doesn't have much of a story to tell. It is a lament I will hear almost every time I visit. Sometimes she even suggests that I should perhaps talk to someone else with a more interesting tale to tell. Even when I ask about her experience as an *ikebana* teacher, for which she has master status, Chizu suggests that there are others, her teacher for one, who are more knowledgeable than she in the art of Japanese flower arranging.

Such statements are *enryo*, the Japanese act of humility in which one dismisses one's importance, needs and/or desires. It is a trait that my own Okinawan mother has instilled in me all too well. In trying to explain the concept to my own son, I tell him, "You know *enryo* is when someone offers you a cookie and you really want it, but out of politeness you say 'no thank you.'" His response is all American, "Why would I do that?"

Chizu is American, but like most Nisei (second generation Japanese American) she retains much of the culture instilled by her Issei (first generation) parents. Both her mother and father came to the U.S. from the Wakayama prefecture, located in the southwestern region of Japan. It is an area famous for its scenic beauty, mountainous with the presence of virgin forests and a river that runs to a magnificent coastline. With its warm climate, Wakayama is the prefecture where spring comes before anywhere else in Honshu, the largest island of Japan. The region is also known for its historic temples and agriculture that includes fruit, vegetables and flowers. Perhaps the Iwata family brought their love of flowers with them when they immigrated to the United States.

"I wouldn't have had the nerve to come to a different country. They were pioneers," Chizu says proudly.

Though she's not clear of the dates, she believes her father came to the U.S. first to work and then returned to Japan to bring a wife back to California with him. It was an arranged marriage Chizu says, adding that her parents were happy. The family owned and operated a nursery in Mountain View for over fifty years.

They grew chrysanthemums at first, she tells me, and later switched to carnations. Chizu thinks it might be because as a child she was allergic to the pollen from the chrysanthemums. I can't help but wonder if this was the real reason. At another time Chizu tells me that many of the other Japanese American growers switched from chrysanthemums to carnations also.

"Sometimes I forget. Someone asks me how old I am and I think, wait a minute... gee, what year was I born?"

Chizu is the *oneesan*, the eldest sister, in a family of three girls and one boy. She never married, never had any children. "I'm too bossy. I like my ways," she tells me, giving us both a good laugh. Still she says she had "a good growing period compared to some Japanese girls," especially since she had a career in the family's nursery business.

She is thankful that she is healthy, telling me the only surgery she ever had was a tonsillectomy as a child. "I always brag to the family, I'm the only one that has everything I was born with"—with the exception of her tonsils, of course.

She turns ninety this year and on one occasion, with great clarity, tells me that she was born in Mountain View on April 23, 1915. Another time when I visit she can't remember how old she is. She's good-natured about it and laughs telling me, "Sometimes I forget. Someone asks me how old I am and I think, wait a minute... gee, what year was I born?" She also tells me, almost as if it were a secret, "I think I was born in Japan. I'm not sure, but I have a funny feeling that I was." Chizu's sister-in-law refutes this claim, telling me that Chizu was, in fact, born in Mountain View.

When Chizu doesn't remember things, I often find myself wondering if it is the dementia or the pain in recalling some events, such as her mother's passing at a young age. I try to be delicate in asking her how old she was when she lost her mother.

"I don't remember," she responds. "I remember her though, but I don't remember how old I was." She does remember that after her mother passed away, a cousin came from Japan to help her father raise her and her siblings.

"She took care of the house. She was older than us. My mother's sister's child came from Japan. She came to take care of us, I think. That's what it was," she says, suddenly remembering. "And then she got married in America. I don't know what happened. I think she got divorced or something like that. I can't remember, but they were separated. But she stuck with my father to raise us, which was nice of her."

Many Issei parents insisted that their American-born children study Japanese as well as receive cultural instruction.

Chizu and her brother and sisters grew up in Mountain View, attending the local public schools. She easily remembers that she attended Whitman Grammar School and though the student population was predominately white, Chizu says she never encountered any discrimination. She fondly recalls a favorite teacher.

"Her last name was Donovan, I'm sure. She took a liking to me and my friend and took us to her house and gave us each a Persian cat. Those long-haired cats. She [Chizu's cat] was beautiful," she says, describing the pet's long, blonde fur. Though she can't remember exactly, she believes the cat's name was Japanese. "My family loved animals. We always had cats and dogs."

She tells me of another teacher, one from high school, who invited her and a friend to her home and served them cream puffs. Even after all these years, Chizu exclaims how delicious they were.

Like many Nisei, Chizu went to Japanese school, attending classes after school and even on Saturdays. Many Issei parents insisted that their American-born children study Japanese as well as receive cultural instruction.

"I hated it," Chizu says bluntly. "I think my father just threw money away." I ask if her siblings went as well. "I don't think my brother went very much. He didn't want to go and, you know, he was the only boy, so... you know, my parents weren't too strict with him. That's why I used to pinch him, because I was jealous." She punctuates the word "pinch" and I can almost feel the sharp pull of skin as her eyes narrow. A mischievous spark comes out from behind the polite Nisei-woman demeanor. She laughs. "I hope he doesn't remember those things." Then as if remembering her manners, she adds, "But he's very nice now."

Chizu's sisters no longer live in the area, but her brother is in Los Altos and still comes to visit her regularly. "He comes over in the morning sometimes and asks, 'Hey, you still living?' and I say, 'Yeah, I sure am.'"

Chizu speaks of her brother often with a great deal of affection. She lights up and becomes animated when she tells tales, obviously proud of her baby brother. She does admit though, to being jealous of his privileged status as the only son in a Japanese family.

"He was a brat," she emphasizes the word. "You know Japanese love boys and he was the only one in the family. So he was spoiled rotten."

She tells me how she used to like to go to the bowling alley to watch him and his friends bowl. I ask her if she bowled, but she says "no," giving no explanation why. Still, when her brother took up golf and Chizu took an interest, he did try to teach her.

"He took me one time and then said, 'forget it.' So, I did." I note that Chizu is often complacent, a trait associated with many Japanese. Most Japanese Americans, even if they don't speak Japanese, are all too familiar with the term, *shikata ga nai* (it can't be helped). The saying was often made regarding the internment of Japanese Americans during World War II, when Executive Order 9066 forced all persons of Japanese ancestry to leave the West Coast. Over 100,000 Japanese Americans were interned in crowded, poorly constructed camps behind barbed wire and under the watch of armed guards.

I note that Chizu is often complacent, a trait associated with many Japanese. Most Japanese Americans, even if they don't speak Japanese, are all too familiar with the term, *shikata ga nai* (it can't be helped).

When I ask Chizu where her family was interned she tells me they weren't. I'm confused and though I want to be polite, I have to pursue this all too important, yet delicate subject. I know that for those who underwent the ordeal, the experience was painful and humiliating. Even though a presidential apology and reparations were issued in 1988, the subject is shameful for many older Japanese Americans and even now many are reluctant to talk about the injustice.

"You didn't go to a camp?" I ask her.

"We were lucky," Chizu tells me. "We didn't go."

"You stayed in Mountain View?" I persist.

"Yes." She is adamant.

I wonder if the experience was so painful that she's blocked it out or if it's one of the many things she is unclear about. So, I pursue the questioning a bit more.

"You didn't have to sell your property or anything?

"No, we were very lucky," Chizu repeats. "My father owned the place, you know. He didn't pay rent, so I think that had something to do with it. A lot of Japanese, you know, they grew blueberries, strawberries, things like that. They had to move around." I realize she doesn't understand what I'm talking about. Perhaps she thinks I'm referring to migrant work camps. Then she changes the subject and talks about how all her friends are now scattered and she's sad that they've lost touch.

I learn from Chizu's brother, Roy, that the family actually didn't go to camp. They moved to Denver at that time, thus avoiding government internment. He doesn't offer details and I don't pry. I know that one of the reasons I can't ask the hard questions is because I am speaking to a Japanese elder male. My own cultural upbringing won't allow me to be so impertinent.

Honor your heritage, respect your elders and don't talk back. With your own people, there is a code of ethics that is expected.

I once was with an African American friend when she was moving into a luxury apartment building. The front desk attendant, an older African American man, introduced himself as "Mister Nelson," then proceeded to give my friend detailed instructions on how she should move in. I watched as my friend, a middle-aged, normally very assertive woman, suddenly became passive, listening attentively to Mr. Nelson, simply nodding respectfully as he continued his litany.

As we left the building, she whispered to me, "See, when an older Black person starts lecturing me I turn into a nine-year-old. Yes, Mr. Nelson," she mimicked herself.

We laughed together. I could relate all too well. Though our cultural backgrounds are different, our mothers had raised us the same. Honor your heritage, respect your elders and don't talk back. With your own people, there is a code of ethics that is expected. And while my Japanese manners won't allow me to be the brash journalist that gets to the bottom of a story, my cultural understanding give me an insight into Chizu's life that need no explanation.

Chizu brightens when I use the few Japanese words that I know. She always marvels how good my Japanese is (which it's not), and asks how I know about Japanese holidays and so much about Japanese food. I politely remind her that my mother is from Okinawa and she always expresses astonishment. I ask her if she celebrated both Japanese and American holidays.

She nods. *"Obon and Oshogatsu,"* she states, referring to the Japanese All Souls' Festival and Japanese New Year.

"You have to eat that moldy thing." She wrinkles her nose and I laugh.

"Mochi?" I ask if she is referring to the cakes made from pounded rice.

Though it is eaten year round now, it is a tradition to eat *mochi* as a New Year's food, when it is freshly prepared at community gatherings at *Oshogatsu*. It's a sticky concoction that must be chewed well, quite different from anything most Westerners are used to. My children and I love mochi, even more than their father, who grew up in Japan.

"I like it," Chizu says. "But I don't see how American people can eat that."

I know that she is referring to white people when she uses the term "American." I grew up speaking the same way, even as a person who is half white. I've found many Asians do the same, particularly if they are immigrants. When I was teaching creative writing at juvenile hall I was trying to explain the Japanese American internment experience to a student of Vietnamese descent. "They're like me, Japanese American." I told him. Suddenly another student who had come to this country as a Cambodian refugee, stood up and yelled at me, "You are not American! I am not American! He is not American!" I understood fully what he meant. For many Asians, if you are not white, you are not American. For a young man of color facing possibly twenty years in prison after trying to survive the only way he knew how, perhaps that's why the rules don't apply. Certainly the U.S. government in 1942 did not recognize persons of Japanese descent as Americans when they ordered them to leave the West Coast.

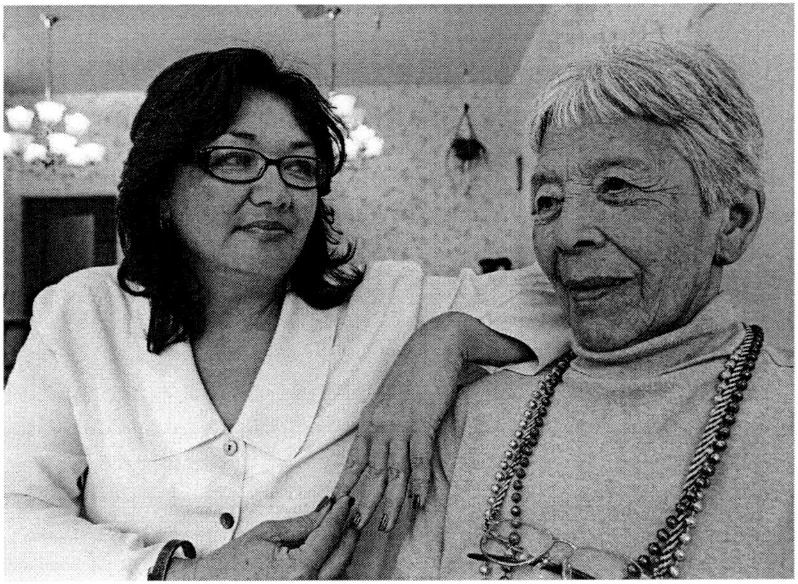

Chizu with her writer, Margaret

After the war, the Iwata family returned to Mountain View and resumed the family nursery business. But it's her recollection of the years before the war that are strongest. She talks fondly of the parties and dances, particularly at the Buddhist Church. I ask if she attended the Buddhist Church in Mountain View.

"Yes, but that was just to play." She smiles and adds, "I didn't learn anything."

I gather from other talks and visits that Chizu seems to have little interest in religion or any subject that requires soul-searching. On one visit, I arrive during dance class. Her dance teacher tells me that Chizu has already had a turn at dancing and suggests that we leave for our visit. Before we get out the door, however, a group of preschool trick-or-treaters arrives for a Halloween celebration, showing off their costumes and singing to the residents of the health center. The women are delighted, and Chizu exclaims over and over again to me, "Aren't they cute!" Once the program is over, an invitation is extended for a worship service that will soon begin. Chizu confers with another woman and they both agree they don't want to go to church. Though she is usually easygoing and willing to participate in most activities, Chizu is adamant about not attending the service. When I ask if she'll sit and talk with me, she thinks I have something to do with church and politely tries to decline. I try to explain that I'm not part of the worship service, but Chizu is confused. I'm ready to give up the visit for the day, but the dance teacher encourages us both to go and talk. Chizu complies. She's fine with me once she understands that I'm not trying to evangelize her.

Perhaps Chizu had not pondered much the teachings of Buddha, but her time at temple obviously offered much in the way of fellowship and culture. When I ask if she enjoyed dancing, referring to the class she just had, Chizu responds enthusiastically. "Yes," she says, "*Obon* dances."

Though I am asking about the dancing that she did just an hour ago, Chizu is remembering *bon odori*, the Japanese dances of the All Souls' Festival. I wonder whether somehow she is making the connection between *Obon* and Halloween, another holiday honoring the dead. *Obon* is a festive celebration held at the end of summer. The temple grounds are decorated with lanterns to light the way for a brief visit from departed ancestors. *Bon odori* is the highlight of the festival when everyone is invited to join in folk dancing to the sound of traditional Japanese music blaring from loudspeakers.

I happily enter her world. "Did you wear kimono?" I ask, then correct myself, "Or, I guess you wore a *yukata*?" The garment is a light, casual version of the formal kimono. Usually it is made of cotton, often in bright colors and festive designs.

Chizu nods. "Yes, *yukata*," she confirms. She tells me that she loved

Obon. "My father made me take lessons," referring to the dance practices held in the weeks preceding the festival.

"We used to go to San Jose when they had their *Obon*. Mountain View, of course, I danced there. We went to Palo Alto even. We traveled around. Some ladies would come to our church too. Mountain View built a beautiful temple. So a lot of out-of-towners used to come to our Obon and dance with us and everything."

"Mountain View built a beautiful temple. So a lot of out-of-towners used to come to our Obon and dance with us and everything."

The talk of *odori* and *yukata* takes Chizu's mind to other kimono moments. I'm sure that as an *ikebana* master, she had to wear a kimono often. "My father bought a lot," she tells me. "You know that belt?"

"The *obi*?" I ask. It is a large cloth belt covering the entire waist from below the breast to almost the hip. The fancy ones are made of silk brocade and are stiff and uncomfortable. One can only sit up straight when wearing an *obi*.

"I couldn't stand that!" Chizu rolls her eyes. "So I tell them, don't tie it tight." Chizu often speaks about the past in the present tense.

We laugh together. "But it's supposed to be tight," I respond.

"Yeah, because it slips down," Chizu shakes her head, smiling. "I look at it now and think, gee, we had a good time."

It is a familiar lament. Chizu frequently reminisces about her friends and how much she misses them. I learn that some of Chizu's father's acquaintances in Japan came to Northern California and also went to work in the flower business. The families kept in touch and the children all grew up together. These are the people that remained Chizu's friends for many years. The past and the present often blur when she talks about them.

"All my friends are scattered. It's a shame in a way. Sometimes at funerals or something we meet each other. But a lot of times I forget their faces. It's so long ago."

Speaking as if he is still alive, she tells me that her family takes the Japanese newspaper so that her father can keep up with the news, especially the obituaries. Having worked at a Japanese American newspaper, I know how important the obituaries are to the Issei and Nisei. Even now, the younger generations, the Sansei and Yonsei, understand the importance of attending funerals, sometimes of people that they hardly even knew.

"Funerals become a gathering time," I comment.

"That's right," Chizu agrees. "You know we're all anxious to see whoever. You know, some of our friends we hadn't seen in ages. And we do meet some of them. Our friends are mutual. You know, we all grew up together, a lot of us in Mountain View."

She speaks fondly and often of her childhood friend Edith, who was her next-door neighbor. "She had brains. Oh god, she was a smart student. I wasn't," Chizu laughs. "I was more of a daydreamer, but somehow or other I got through school. They didn't demote me. Every time I think of those days... it was good times. I loved it." Chizu believes Edith is still alive, living in San Jose. "I'm glad she's still around. You know, some place close. I see her every so often."

I come to know that as much as she loved the art of *ikebana*, the school itself also served as an important part of her social life.

Chizu's other friends are those she met through *ikebana*. Her conversation turns easily to the friendships she made in the Ikenobo School, one of the art's traditional styles of study. I come to know that as much as she loved the art of *ikebana*, the school itself also served as an important part of her social life. She tells me that the meetings drew people from all over the Bay Area and beyond. Trying to get an idea how large the gatherings were, I ask how many attended the meetings.

"Were there maybe twenty-five, fifty people in your *ikebana* group?"

"Oh, more than that!" Chizu exclaims. She easily rattles off a list of the places that members came from: "Oakland, Sacramento sometimes, Monterey, Watsonville, San Jose..."

"So, you might have a hundred people?" I ask.

"Oh yeah," she says. "Over [a hundred], I think. And it's nice; the head

北 加 支 部

Ikenobo Ikebana Society of Northern California Chapter

925 Wright Ave., Mountain View, CA94043

TEL (650)968-3206

支部長 岩田千鶴

副支部長 佐伯欣水

リセージ・欣子

会計 小畑るり子

末政翠竹

書記(日) 中村千津子

書記(英) メタクサス・英子

会史係 中野玉枝

会計監査 俣野翠雲

松本千代子

顧問 澤井村代

佐伯進

外支部員一同

Chizu was president of the society from 1996-1999

of the school has different teachers come. It's the same style, but something is different from each of the teachings. You learn more. We're very fortunate to have a chapter in San Francisco. Sometimes people from Washington State come to our chapter and we get ideas from them too. Everyone has different ideas. We make a lot of friends. Otherwise, we wouldn't know these people."

Chizu talks as if it were still part of her life. Then suddenly, she seems to realize that her *ikebana* memories are something from the past, but she's not sure quite how long ago. "That was the Ikenobo School. We used to have fun. But now, everybody has children and they have to go to school and this and that, so I don't see them so much, which is a shame."

Chizu is petite, very pretty and very feminine. Her snow-white hair, cropped short, is neatly combed and her nails are always manicured.

It seems flowers were always a part of Chizu's life. From a young age she "bunched carnations" for the market and worked in the family nursery well into her adult years. As a young girl she began studying *ikebana,* going on to become a master teacher.

"I was a tomboy," Chizu tells me as if it is a confession. "So my father made me go to *ikebana* school thinking maybe I could be more ladylike. But it didn't work."

We laugh and I ask, "You stayed a tomboy?"

"Yeah, I liked to play baseball and things like that."

I try to picture her as a tomboy, but it doesn't quite fit. Chizu is petite, very pretty and very feminine. Her snow-white hair, cropped short, is neatly combed and her nails are always manicured. Though she dresses casually, often in sweats, she usually wears pastels or other soft colors. She's often adorned in plastic necklaces.

When I bring *ikebana* books to share with her, Chizu is confident in her knowledge of the art. It's clear she's an authority. Despite her difficulty in recalling the past, she easily names all the flowers in the books, the tools, techniques and the different schools of *ikebana.* She tells me that originally it was the priests who taught *ikebana* and I learn that the art is much more than flower arranging. It is a moving meditation and a spiritual interpretation of nature.

Chizu explains to me the principles of *shin, so, tai,* the three elements of the art which all schools of *ikebana* embrace. *Shin,* the strongest and often longest element in the composition, is seen as a symbol of man's attainment of enlightenment. *So,* the supporting branch, symbolizes man situated between

"The people in Japan, they wanted to meet me because my mother had me first. I had a brother and sisters, but they wanted to see *me*."

heaven and earth. And *tai*, the smallest and shortest segment of the arrangement, is representative of earth.

We are looking over the books in the activity room in the Alzheimer's unit of the nursing home. Chizu seems oblivious to the goings-on about the room. The radio blares R. Kelly's "I Believe I Can Fly." One woman goes into a coughing fit; another recites the Hail Mary over and over again. An attendant comes in and affectionately joins in the recitation. Three men sit at a round table and the attendant greets them, wheeling one closer to the table, then setting some toys in front of them. One fumbles with the colorful plastic puzzle tubes that look like baby toys. The others stare vacantly out the window or into empty space.

Despite the noise that I find distracting, Chizu continues paging through the books, obviously delighting in the different designs. I ask if the viewing of *ikebana* is supposed to be inspiring.

"Yeah, it's *supposed* to," she mutters. We both laugh.

"I just glance at it, but I think each stem has some kind of meaning. You know, my father sent me to Japanese school, but I didn't pay too much attention. And I'm sorry I did that because after I started *ikebana* that could have helped me more, if I had paid more attention."

"To the language you mean?" I ask. "Uh huh. That's one of my regrets." It is not the first time Chizu has admonished herself for not being more knowledgeable about Japanese. She admits on more than one occasion that she is ashamed of her "broken Japanese."

"The people in Japan, they wanted to meet me because my mother had me first. I had a brother and sisters, but they wanted to see *me*." I detect an uncharacteristic tone of pride in this statement, unlike the sense of *enryo* that I have so often observed in Chizu. "So, finally my father sent me to Japan and I met those Japanese cousins and aunties. But, my Japanese wasn't too fluent, so I think they were disappointed."

Chizu is confused about how often she's been to Japan, but from what I can decipher from different accounts, she visited her parents' homeland a number of times. As an adult, Chizu went to Japan with the Ikenobo School of San Francisco, traveling to Kyoto and studying the art there. Again, what she remembers most is the difficulty with the language. I've encountered many other Japanese Americans who found visiting Japan stressful because they are perceived as Japanese, yet they are American.

"Not that I don't like it," she says about visiting Japan again. "But, I don't want to go back."

I understand. Because I don't look fully Japanese, when I visit Japan I am treated as a *gaijin* (a foreigner), and people are usually friendly and polite. They don't expect me to bow or use *ohashi* (chopsticks) or to speak Japanese, and when I do they praise me. The expectations for *gaijin* are much lower. It's no wonder so many Westerners love Japan. Chizu and I talk about how Westerners so often know more about Japan and Japanese culture than we do.

Because I don't look fully Japanese, when I visit Japan I am treated as a *gaijin* (a foreigner), and people are usually friendly and polite.

"Sometimes Caucasians catch on much faster than Japanese," Chizu says of those that study *ikebana*.

I tell her I've found the same in the Japanese language classes I've taken.

"Japanese, you know, we think we know it all," she says and we both laugh.

Spotting a photo of *ikebana* scissors in a book, she proceeds to tell me about the special technique in using them. The thought takes her back in time again.

"Now that I think about it, where's my scissors? Oh god," she frets, worrying that she's lost them. "I think they're quite expensive now."

Chizu's memory frequently plays these tricks. On another visit, we talk about another favorite subject of hers, cars. She is telling me about the cars she owned, always Buicks, when suddenly she is somewhere else.

"Now that we speak of the car, I wonder where I parked it." She consoles herself saying, "I have some American friend with me, so she'll know, 'cause I gave her a ride." She returns abruptly to the present to admonish herself for her memory loss: "Oh, what a sad case."

Apparently Chizu loved to drive and was often the driver for her *ikebana* group.

"My friends didn't drive. They didn't have cars, so any meetings or parties, I drove."

In Chizu's generation, many Nisei women never learned to drive. Chizu seems rather proud of her accomplishment. She says she learned to drive quite young, perhaps before she was of legal age.

"My father always had a car. I don't know how he did it, it must have cost a penny." She explains the phrase to me. "You know, a lot of money."

"All the policemen knew my father because he loved to drink and they liked to drink sake too. You know when I come to think of it, it's a wonder they got away like that."

She tells me that her father liked to drink, which is why she learned to drive when she was so young. That way she could drive her father around if he'd been drinking. "You know I didn't want us to get killed or anything," she says quite seriously. I try to keep from laughing.

She recalls a friend of her father who sold Buicks: "He liked my father. He used to come to the house all the time. So, I always drove a Buick. I still do. It was not a convertible, [it was] a sedan, a small one. I just love that car. I had a black one. I think I was partial to black." Her memory skips again. "Gee, I forgot what I'm driving now. It's still black."

The conversation about cars takes us back to the days of prohibition and her father's drinking. Chizu was a teenager at the time and says she remembers that a Japanese man in San Jose used to make sake and deliver it late at night.

"I remember those things. My brother [and sisters], they don't. I remember them delivering it at midnight. But there were some cops who knew about it. So the man that made the sake, he bribed them. So, they'd come over when that man came to deliver the sake to my father. The policemen used to take the sake. So, you know, that's why I got my license when I was not supposed to. That's why I drove. All the policemen knew my father because he loved to drink and they liked to drink sake too. You know when I come to think of it, it's a wonder they got away like that."

I enjoy the story and feel privileged that she chooses to share her family secret with me. She may not remember me the next time I visit, but each time we meet, we somehow bond. This is one of those moments.

The next time I visit Chizu she is sleeping. She has told me before that she is often sleepy, that she likes to sleep—another thing we have in common. I find her asleep in her wheelchair in the activity room. One woman rolls her wheelchair back and forth against a table. I wonder if I should offer to help her move away from the table, then suddenly realize that she may not be trying to go anywhere. She just needs to move. It seems to be a kind of stressful pacing, only this pacing is done in a wheelchair.

There is an empty chair next to Chizu, so I sit there and lightly touch her on the arm. She drowsily opens her eyes. I greet her, reminding her who I am. She's polite, but I know she doesn't recognize me. I ask her how she is; she answers, "sleepy." She agrees to let me just sit with her for a bit.

Carol, the activities director, arrives and pulls up a chair across from the group of women lined up against the wall. She brings a new energy to the room as she holds up a book and announces that she will be reading from *Don't Sweat the Small Stuff*. After greeting everyone, she reads a passage about letting go of stubbornness. She talks about her own tendency toward stubbornness and asks the women one by one what they are inflexible about. Some deny having such a streak. Another declares she isn't stubborn, just obstinate. Chizu laughs with the others, but declines to admit any such trait of her own.

Kindly including me in the discussion, Carol asks what I am stubborn about. I readily volunteer that I expect too much of people. She consoles me, admitting that she used to be that way, but has mellowed as she aged. "Maybe there is hope for me after all," I think to myself. Suddenly I realize that I'm enjoying being a part of this group of white-haired women that once seemed so far from my own reality.

Suddenly I realize that I'm enjoying being a part of this group of white-haired women that once seemed so far from my own reality.

Carol continues to talk about how we are all opinionated. To my surprise, Chizu heartily agrees with her. I have rarely heard Chizu express an opinion about anything, something I've attributed to her "Nisei-ness"—the need to be polite and noncontroversial. Once again, I realize, I'm stereotyping.

The woman at the table continues to roll back and forth frantically in her wheelchair until Carol addresses her: "Alice, come over here and join us." Alice starts to protest, but Carol, reaching out with a strong arm, pulls Alice's chair close to her and gently takes her hand. Alice beams, completely unselfconscious of her missing teeth. This is a beautiful woman, I realize. Despite the mottled, wrinkled skin, missing teeth and thinning white hair, Alice is radiant when she smiles. She kneads Carol's hands in hers as Carol continues the discussion.

When Carol announces that it's time for exercise class, I decide to leave. The women all laugh, undoubtedly thinking that I'm lazy, which isn't too off base. I tell Chizu that on my next visit I'll bring flowers so that she might give me an *ikebana* lesson. As I go out the door, she reminds me not to forget to bring leaves.

The next time I visit, I bring leaves as well as flowers, vases and *kenzan* or what Chizu refers to as a "frog pin," to stick the flowers into. Chizu is in art class and Sharon, the art teacher, graciously allows me to have her put aside her watercolor painting to do an arrangement during her class. Chizu and the others in the class exclaim over the purple iris, yellow tulips and orange coffee bean blossoms I've brought. Fortunately, the Korean woman who owns the flower shop knows a bit about flower arranging herself and has advised me on my selection.

As Chizu begins the first composition, Sharon asks her to talk about her thought process in creating the arrangement. Chizu simply sighs, as if even contemplating such a question tires her. "I just look at it and I just put the flower there," she says with a laugh.

"Fair enough," Sharon says, respectful of an artist's mood.

I am reminded of a time when I interviewed another Japanese artist. The woman's medium was "found objects," so I asked what inspired her creations. She told me that she didn't like to think about it too much because she felt the thought processes interfered with creativity. I didn't know what to ask her after that.

Chizu gives little instruction about the flower-arranging process, but considerately asks about my preferences. I become her assistant, cutting branches, flowers and leaves at her instruction as she casually finds a place for them in the *kenzan*. Though she seems not to contemplate the composition as she works, the arrangement unfolds beautifully. She makes adjustments easily.

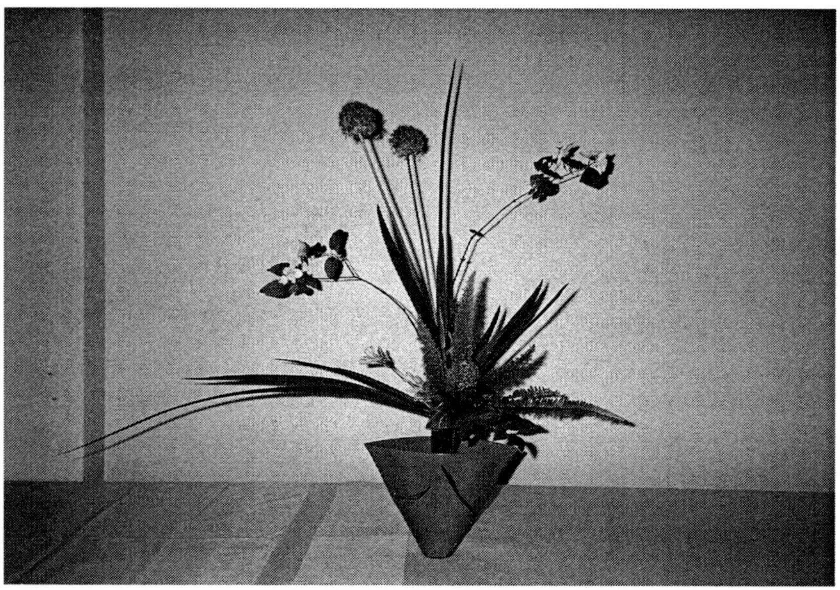

Chizu's floral art, 1995

"Wait a minute," she tells me before I cut a flower. "I'm going to lift this up, the leaf." And she gently pushes up the leaf around a tulip. I'm amazed. I never would have thought to rearrange a flower's leaf. I didn't even know it was possible, but once the stem is trimmed, the leaf slides up easily, making room for another flower. One of the principles in *ikebana* is that nothing should compete for attention.

She instructs me to cut a long-stemmed iris very short and I do so with some trepidation. With quiet confidence, Chizu pulls the arrangement together. The result is a striking array of tall, varied greens framing a soft yellow tulip that drapes to one side. A short shock of purple—the iris that I've just cut—completes the composition.

Chizu's friend across the table from her prods her on. "You're doing a good job, honey."

"You think so?" Chizu counters, good-naturedly.

It takes her a short time to create two beautiful arrangements. She gives some consideration to how long the arrangement will be on display, telling me that the blooms will open up later and add more contrast to the composition. When she is finished she simply tells me, "I don't think we should put any more in." We all admire the compositions, marveling over their elegance and simplicity. We talk about naming the two arrangements.

"You name it." Chizu suggests, giving me the honor of giving a title to the piece, a practice in Japanese art. I'm at a loss, as is everyone else in the room. Chizu refuses to name the pieces herself, and we leave them unnamed.

Chizu asks me my favorite and I choose the one with the short iris. "It fits this vase," she notes. She compliments my choice of flowers, telling me I have good taste.

"Thank you," I tell her. "But, *you* brought it to life.

One beautiful flower that no one knows the name of is left and Chizu worries what we should do with it. I urge her to keep it. At first she hesitates, but finally agrees, telling me she'll put it on her *butsudan*, the family altar that so many Japanese families have in their home. I'm sure she doesn't have a *butsudan* in her room at the healthcare center, but I know that in her mind, there is a place for the flower beside a bowl of rice and cup of sake that she keeps there as an offering.

I'm sure she doesn't have a *butsudan* in her room at the healthcare center, but I know that in her mind, there is a place for the flower beside a bowl of rice and cup of sake that she keeps there as an offering.

Although Chizu clearly enjoys the ikebana experience, she sends me off with the arrangements when I leave, reminding me to water the flowers.

Sharon tries once again to engage Chizu in her creative process: "So any last words you have about your beautiful art piece?"

"No, no." Chizu is adamant. "I think it came out real nice" is all she offers. Then, in her usual humble manner, she seeks to avoid the recognition: "The materials are good."

When I have to leave, Chizu simply smiles and goes back to her watercolor. How very Zen, I think. She enjoys the creative process and is not attached to the final outcome.

I remember her telling me when we talked another time that flowers were her only hobby. "I didn't have other hobbies. I didn't play golf or anything. I turned to flowers." Though one may wonder if flowers became her way of life simply because it was the family business, I believe Chizu was born to the way of flowers. Watching her in the art of ikebana, I understand that flowers were more than a hobby—they were a passion.

Though one may wonder if flowers became her way of life simply because it was the family business, I believe Chizu was born to the way of flowers.

I feel honored to bring the displays home and proudly tell my family that the arrangements are the work of an *ikebana* master. Their harmonious beauty graces my home for a week before they begin to wilt and I am sad when I have to throw the flowers away.

I've come to think of my visits with Chizu much like *ikebana*. Every meeting is new, just like every flower arrangement. The beauty is in the moment of creation. And like flowers that begin to die as soon as they are picked, my visits with Chizu will fade from her memory as soon as I leave. Yet, at the moment of our visits, we share beauty through our laughter, for we always laugh when we visit together.

At the end of one of our meetings, Chizu asks me if I have my car. I tell her I do. She asks if I could drop her off in Mountain View. I pause, realizing that she wants me to take her to her home on Wright Avenue, and I respond, "I'll take you back to your room." She accepts my offer and as we walk back together down the hall with Chizu alongside me scooting her wheelchair with her feet, she tells me she's not sure of the way.

"I think we turn left," I tell her and add in Japanese, *"Hidari."*

Chizu brightens at the word and repeats it. *"Hidari."* And we turn left together down the corridor, back to her room. ■

WRITER'S PROFILE

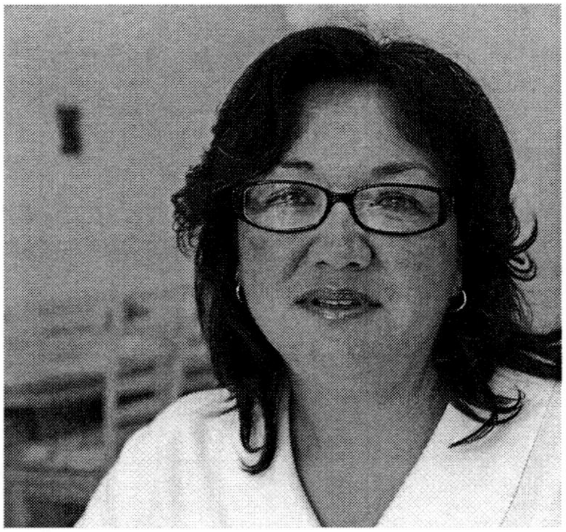

Margaret S.A. Bacon

I was born in Okinawa, and growing up as a hapa of Okinawan, English, Irish, Scottish, and French descent in predominately white Orange County, I had little contact with the Japanese American community. It wasn't until moving to San Francisco as an adult that I even learned of the World War II incarceration of Japanese Americans. In fact, the concept of a Japanese American culture, apart from Japanese culture, was foreign to me.

It was through elders that I came to know the Japanese American community. In the early '80s I took a part time job driving for Kimochi, Inc., the Japanese American senior service organization located in San Francisco's Japantown. It was the perfect day job while I wrote short stories and worked on a children's novel (or so I tell myself that's what I was doing). I got to practice my Japanese on the patient and appreciative Issei (first generation Japanese Americans), learned to navigate my way around the city, and ate the most delicious "senior" lunches. It was because of the invitation of one of my passengers to the annual chicken teriyaki bazaar at a local Japanese American church that my husband and I became members of Pine United Methodist Church.

The Japanese American community also provided me with my first professional writing job. For two years I served as the English Editorial Assistant at the Hokubei Mainichi, a bilingual daily located in the heart of Japantown. I've since gone on to write for a few other Japanese American publications and currently serve on the board of two community magazines.

In between part-time jobs to support my writing habit, I'm always working on a novel or two, sometimes simultaneously. I've got a feeling I don't choose so much to write as it chooses me.

SYDNEY KOSSEN

Reutlinger Community for Jewish Living
Danville, California
with
Michele Bigley

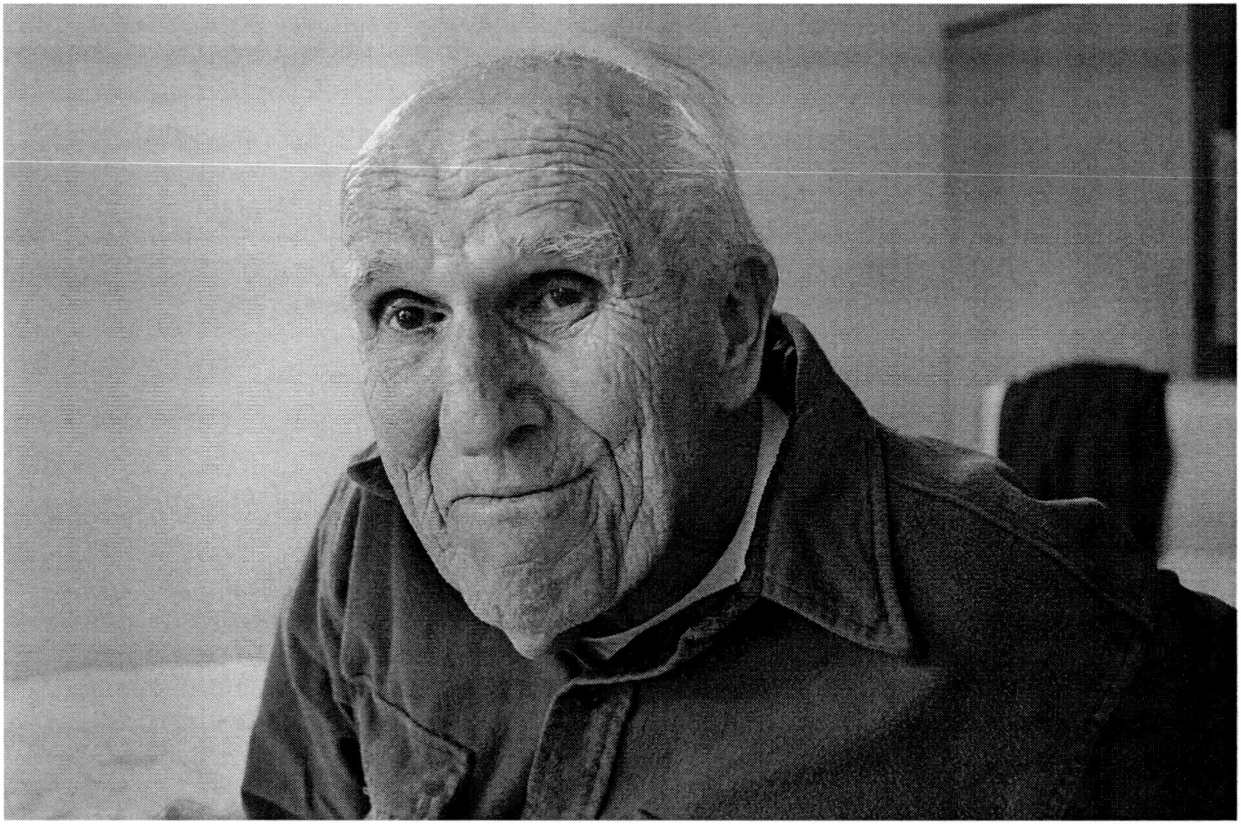

"There is joy in looking back"

In the center of the wall is a black-and-white photo. Maybe thirty years old, Sydney Kossen leans against an old car; his pressed suit rides up, showing off thin, agile ankles; a fedora hangs over his full head of hair, slightly covering his left eye. His wife stands next to him, swanlike, in a stylish dress. He grins as though anything and everything will be possible.

For Sydney, anything was possible.

He was the first Jewish editor of the University of Washington newspaper; the man whom Willie Brown deemed the "Dean of Northern California Political Writers"; who, despite the protests of his loved ones, went to fight in World War II; who, despite hearing and vision impairments, became a well-known journalist; a man who wasn't afraid of presidents, senators, governors or love. Sydney Kossen never took no for an answer.

Today, Sydney lives in the Reutlinger Community for Jewish Living. Thirty-nine miles from San Francisco: the city where he spent his adult life, the city he wrote about, where he met and married his wife, owned a house, and raised children. Now, Sydney's days are quiet. They consist of conversations with nurses and doctors, the rabbi, residents; telephone calls to his wife Jeanette; Corn Flakes, coffee, Kosher food; the morning news read to him from his rival paper—the San Francisco Chronicle; classical music. Jeanette visits on Mondays, occasionally with their son. Sometimes there are entertainers. But mostly, Sydney lies in bed and remembers.

I approached the vinyl chair that would become a place of comfort for me through the next six months and wondered how I could possible do justice in my tribute to this man—
a professional interviewer and Reutlinger's favorite resident.

When I first met Sydney Kossen, he wore navy sweatpants, a Washington sweatshirt and thick glasses despite the sweltering July heat outside. He inched his walker to the windowed side of the room and told me to take a seat. I repeated a bit louder that I was interested in his life; that I wanted to write a story about him. He suddenly appeared boyish and excited, admitting how flattered he was to be chosen for the project, then directing me to look at an article taped on the wall near his bed—the only decoration in the white room, save a few recent photos of him and his son and a pink handmade afghan on his single bed. The article was a tribute to his work as a political journalist, with excerpts from his interviews with Pat Brown, Ronald Reagan and David Ben Gurion. Attached was a photo of him, maybe twenty years younger, his face wrinkled with pride. I approached the vinyl chair that would become a place of comfort for me through the next six months and wondered how I could possible do justice in my tribute to this man—a professional interviewer and Reutlinger's favorite resident. I was a mere twenty-nine-year-old graduate student, wanting to understand the agedness that I will encounter, that my grandparents experienced, that my parents cautiously approached.

I began firing questions at him—"Where were you born? Where is your family from? What were your parents' names?"—hardly awaiting his answers. It was in my haste to learn more about this man, to make him comfortable talking to me and me with him, that I realized how fast and unprepared I was. Like most relationships I cultivated as a twenty-something, I felt rushed to know all the specifics of his past so we could get to the heart of his existence, to his loves, his passions, his fears. To a place of trust that we young people so crave in our communications with each other. But Sydney's room was an unhurried oasis, one so different from that which I encountered each day in San Francisco. Most of my day was spent rushing from one appointment to the next, checking e-mails and cell phones, driving over the speed limit to get to my destination faster, gobbling down my food, multitasking. Here I was now, sitting in a room with a man whose thoughts marinated before releasing; where gaps in the conversation made me ask and re-ask the same questions for fear he could not understand my rushed vocabulary. I tried to remind myself to breathe, to remember the reasons why I was here, but outside the room I heard someone cough, someone else calling for a nurse, and I couldn't recall one reason.

The next Wednesday, after a pep talk from a septuagenarian friend, I arrived with lists of questions and a tape recorder, ready to capture the intricacies of Sydney's slow speech and methodical nature. He seemed a bit more at ease and without much prodding began telling the story of his parents—Orthodox Jews from northern Russia, not far from Leningrad, not far from my great-grandparents' homes. This was the turn of the century, when Jews were being rounded up, exploited, kidnapped and killed. Sydney's grandfather had recently fought and died for the Russian army and his grandmother didn't want any more of the family to die for the tsar, so she instructed Sydney's father, Harry, to go to the United States. Understanding that he could not own land unless he followed his father's footsteps into war, Harry left his wife Sadie with their two surviving children—Jack and Rose—and took a boat to the United States.

He was a blacksmith looking for opportunity. With the help of the Jewish Immigration Society, Harry found a job at the Studebaker plant in South Bend, Indiana, where he spent his days making carriages. But the Homestead Act lured him farther west. After reading an article in the Jewish newspaper, Harry realized he could claim a 160-acre parcel of land for just an $18 filing fee. That day, he hopped a train to western Washington to purchase his homestead. Harry then sent for Sadie and the children.

After a few years, they sold their homestead and got a flat in the east side of Seattle—in a low-income Jewish neighborhood. Sadie and Harry were refreshed to be in a city, near a synagogue and people who spoke Yiddish, near butcher shops and fruit stands, where they weren't constantly covered with dirt. Sadie's spirits lifted, and before long, Sadie gave birth to Carl. Then on October 24, 1915, Sydney was born. He was the seventh and last child.

"The baby." Sydney said with an ironic grin.

Sydney's mother gave him the Jewish name Shimon, or Simon, in English. But his eldest sister Rose didn't want him to be called Simon; she thought kids would tease him by calling him "Simple Simon."

Sydney's mother gave him the Jewish name Shimon, or Simon, in English. But his eldest sister Rose didn't want him to be called Simon; she thought kids would tease him by calling him "Simple Simon." So she changed his name to Sydney. Then in his first grade class, there were two children named Sydney; his teacher pointed at the youthful, short-panted Sydney Kossen, the man who would later have his name in print daily, and said, "You will be the S-Y Sydney [not S-I Sidney]." As Sydney explained, "It stuck."

Sydney's brothers and sisters helped his mother look after him, but it was Rose who took most of the responsibility. "My sister Rose was disappointed that I wasn't a girl. She wanted a little sister, but I couldn't have had a better big sister," Sydney added. Though she had her own children to care for, she helped Sadie prepare Kosher dinners, often trying out kugels and casseroles she learned at the cooking classes at the Jewish Community Center. The children would say, "Ma, you never made this before,"' and Sadie, always ready to give credit to her children, said, "Teresa [Rose's Yiddish name] showed me this."

Sydney laughed when he explained that Rose's oldest son, who was only five years younger than Sydney, used to call Sydney's mother "Ma." But his laughter turned to seriousness: "He died sometime ago. I am the last of the kids."

Sydney recalled how, after dinners, the family would watch Jack Benny

Sydney recalled how, after dinners, the family would watch Jack Benny on the fuzzy television and how Harry would have to "whop the television on the side to get a good picture."

on the fuzzy television and how Harry would have to "whop the television on the side to get a good picture." Relating this, Sydney laughed boyishly. I imagined that it was the same chuckle he had as a child, sitting Indian-style on the rug before the TV, watching his father curse and beat up the television after a long day's work at the blacksmith shop. I imagined that his father would smell like oil, even though he had washed himself before dinner; that his mother would nag Harry to stop hitting the television or he would break it; that the children would be giggling into their pajama tops. But none of this Sydney said. He just laughed like the child he once was, now framed by the picture window in his room, with the giant leaves of the magnolia tree behind him.

On my next visit, Sydney recalled one of his clearest memories—the day he became a man. Even though Sydney was still forced to attend his mostly Jewish high school in eastern Seattle, the day he was called to the Torah signified adulthood. That morning, Sydney wore Jack's old suit that was still a little too big. The sleeves swung around his knuckles. A belt pulled the pants up to his ribs so that the bottoms would not drag on the cement as Harry led Sydney down the path to manhood. They passed the pines, the flats, Sydney's elementary school, then his high school, the children he had grown up playing stickball with, all in silence, understanding that something was supposed to change on that day. And it did. At the synagogue, Sydney was called to the Torah. Though Sydney does not remember what he read that day, I hope he read about his namesake, Shimon, or his favorite Jewish legend, Moses, or maybe he read the story of Yahweh, who first inscribed letters onto stone for communication with God.

With his bar mitzvah and high school completed, Sydney went to work as a blacksmith's helper at the truck-body business of his father's ex-partner. But when Harry found out that Sydney was not getting the National Recovery Administration (NRA) minimum of $14.50 a week, he marched down to the shop demanding a raise for his son. Eventually, the government forced Sydney's boss to pay him his back wages—$282.32. On the recommendation of a friend, Sadie suggested he deposit his riches in the University National Bank, on the University of Washington campus. It was a suggestion that would change his life.

Sydney had never seen anything like a university campus—sprawling with trees and grassy fields, full of students walking so purposefully past Denny Hall, a palace of a building with its columns and windows. The scene was so impressive that he enrolled immediately. On his first day of college, Sydney recalled, "I was awed, excited, so glad and proud to be there." His quick wit and compassion led him to make friends immediately. These contemporaries guided him through the trials of early college life. He majored in engineering because he thought he would be more successful. "I wanted to please my father—even though he thought that route would be too hard for me," admitted Sydney. He thought that because of his experience in machine shops that he would do well. It took a year for Sydney to realize that mechanical engineering wasn't for him, so he volunteered to write articles for the school newspaper. Writing his first college-level piece convinced him to change his major to journalism. He covered science, liberal arts, and even the engineering beats; he won a scholarship to a convention in Canada, kept a B average, and became a member of the honorary journalist society Sigma Delta Chi.

"I was the first Jewish editor of the University of Washington newspaper," Sydney added, a tinge of pride in his voice.

After college, he took a job at the International News Service (INS) as a correspondent for the Seattle Post, moving on at twenty-two to find a position in Sacramento, California, as a reporter. He worked on the newswire, covering the state beat— public works, accidents—whatever the editor told him to report. He was excited to get paid to write. That was when Sydney began developing the voice he would later be respected for: one of specificity, honesty and integrity.

When a job in the San Francisco bureau of the International News Service opened up in the mid-'30s, he

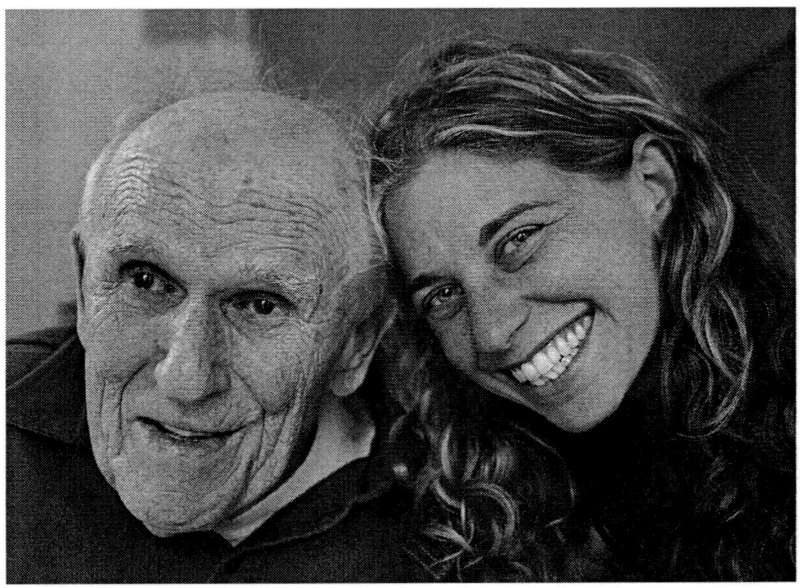

Sydney with his writer, Michele

snapped it up. Fogtown was like nothing he had ever seen before—the fingers of fog reaching over the hills, kissing the bay, yet not entirely hiding the buildings or bridges. He knew this would become home.

It was during that time, when he worked the wires for the INS, that Sydney started frequenting the social activities at the Jewish Community Center. On a chilly summer day, he was in the lounge talking to some friends about the war when a doe-eyed girl with wet brown hair walked into the room. She carried a bag with a damp bathing suit and had the flushed cheeks of someone who had just exercised—a flush that made Sydney's heart race. Who was this girl? he wondered, asking every man in his circle. Until one shrugged, "That's Jeanette. She went to Cal and teaches religious school at Temple Emanuel."

That's all Sydney needed to know. He walked right up to that girl and, within a few dates, knew she would be his wife. She was everything he wanted in a partner: a nice Jewish girl who, along with being a Hebrew school teacher, taught in Tracy because there weren't any openings in San Francisco; she was determined, strong, beautiful, filling his mind with her picture, her slow sweet voice, her laugh. While she was away, Sydney would work long hours, and when she would come home on the weekends, he would use his earnings to take her on dates—Italian dinners in North Beach, movies, walks up Twin Peaks.

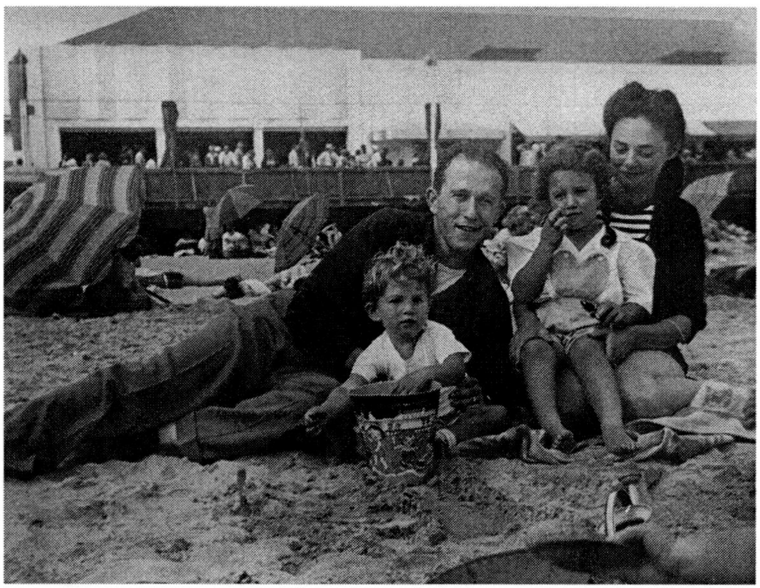

The Kossen family in Santa Cruz, 1946

Marriage came along later. The wedding was at her Uncle Jake's house in Sea Cliff. Sydney's family could not attend the celebration, so Sydney made the photographer take plenty of pictures of his stunning new wife—in her white floral gown, lightly painted cheeks, and wispy hair drawn up out of her face. She looked ethereal. And Sydney could not have been prouder in his newly fitted suit, ready to commit to this woman for the rest of his life.

They honeymooned in Seattle. Jeanette was nervous because she didn't speak Russian and her family was not as religious as Sydney's. She was afraid that they would not accept her. Proud Sydney kept reminding her that they would love her as much as he did. And it was the truth. His mother, pleased with the fact that Jeanette was a religious school teacher, accepted her into the Kossen clan with a warm hug and, since it was the Sabbath, a feast of roasted chicken and potatoes.

"It was exciting when she [Barbara] was born. She was the apple of my eye."

During the early years of their marriage, Sydney and Jeanette lived on 14th Avenue and Balboa. He continued working at the International News Service, spending his days reporting on the war and the growing tensions in Europe and Asia. Jeanette finally got a teaching job as a substitute in San Francisco. And soon after, they had their first child, Barbara. "It was exciting when she was born. She was the apple of my eye. At night I would hurry home and take her out for a walk in her stroller." I pictured Sydney, showing his beautiful little angel off to the neighbors. For Sydney, "being a parent is the greatest pleasure in life."

But his greatest pleasure was cut short too soon. When Jeanette was pregnant with their second child, Michael, Sydney learned that he was about to be drafted for the army. He took the navy officer's exam. "I joined the navy before the army could get me," he explains. Jeanette didn't think it was necessary because not everyone was drafted. She suspected he was volunteering because of the news he heard over the wires—of concentration camps and the extermination of the Jews. Perhaps it was out of national pride or a need to be like his grandfather. She tried to stop him and reminded him that they needed him here, at home; reminded him that she was pregnant and that they had a toddler. But when Sydney made up his mind, there was no debating. He boarded a train for New York as a naval officer—the start of five years at sea.

The next Wednesday we were to meet, Sydney was late. He was talking with the rabbi and did not want to be disturbed. I waited in the Danville sun and began to realize how much I looked forward to these visits. Not only did I have the opportunity to go back in time whenever I walked through the doors of this care center, but talking to Sydney slowed me down, reminded me of what was important. The miniscule details of the past, the unreturned phone calls, the slights by family members or friends, the lovers' spats, didn't make it into Sydney's recounting of the important events of his life. What mattered were the births, the deaths, the loves, marriage, faith, respect. That was life.

When I returned to the center, Sydney and I took our regular seats in his room. Remembering where we left off, Sydney explained that other than the pride of fighting for his country and his people, he received another "souvenir" from World War II—his hearing and vision were permanently impaired by naval gunfire. At first, it was merely a ringing in the ears, then later he would be unable to hear his wife's voice in his right ear. As for his sight, he would wear glasses until the winter of his years, when he would become legally blind.

"No [California politician] had a longer career as a smear artist than Richard Nixon... He gave dirty politics a bad name," he [Sydney] wrote.

Through these challenges, Sydney almost enjoyed being a soldier. As a gunnery officer, he felt like one of the boys, a part of a team of men coming together to experience the joy of the Asian sea. The florescent sunrises and sunsets, flying fish, traveling whales, playful dolphins, the rocking of the cots to lull him to sleep no matter what time. Missing his family, he took the position as a father figure to the younger soldiers. He inspired the teenagers to get their diplomas through the armed forces extension courses. He told them that if they didn't graduate from high school, they would have a hard time finding jobs. Then he made a deal with his crew: if they signed up for classes, he would help them with their lessons. Thanks to Sydney, all his soldiers graduated from high school while they sailed across the Pacific.

But a far more difficult job awaited Sydney and his fellow soldiers at the end of their voyage: to fight for their country. They would "take over the small islands and clear out the Japanese," securing island after island. One afternoon, after the crew of two hundred had completed a mission, Kamikazes flew toward their ship. They could hear the sound of the plane descending in the distance and knew it was coming straight for them. Scared, but needing to be the voice of power and reason, Sydney ordered his boys to shoot them down.

While Sydney was in the navy, Jeanette served as the Kossen family officer on land. Alone with two young children, she bought a house on 33rd Avenue in the Sunset District of San Francisco. She learned to care for her children and herself with strength unique to the women who were left behind during the days of war. Five-year-old Michael had only met his father on a few occasions when Sydney returned home from the war.

Shortly after, Sydney's career took off. He worked for the *San Francisco*

News for three years as a rewrite man, then went to the *Examiner*, where he covered politics for twelve years before becoming the political editor. He traveled to Sacramento, Washington DC, Europe, Israel and Asia to attend political conventions, press conferences and delegations. He never shied away from telling the truth and was never afraid to challenge the people in power—it was a stance that didn't always leave him with a big fan base.

There was the state senator from Sacramento who didn't like Sydney's opinion of his politics, so the senator tried to punch Sydney in the nose. Being the true journalist that he was, Sydney phoned that event right into the news desk and they made a page one story about it. Another time, Sydney told a columnist that two San Francisco assemblymen were "the City's equivalent of Tweedle-Dee and Tweedle-Dumb." When the columnist used Sydney's description of the politicians in his article, one of the assemblymen approached Sydney with a gruff, "What's this Tweedle-Shit?" Always the man of grace, Sydney replied, "I don't tell the columnists what to write; I just give them the news." The assemblyman stormed off, leaving Sydney proud that he could "educate a politician, even if it was in a small way."

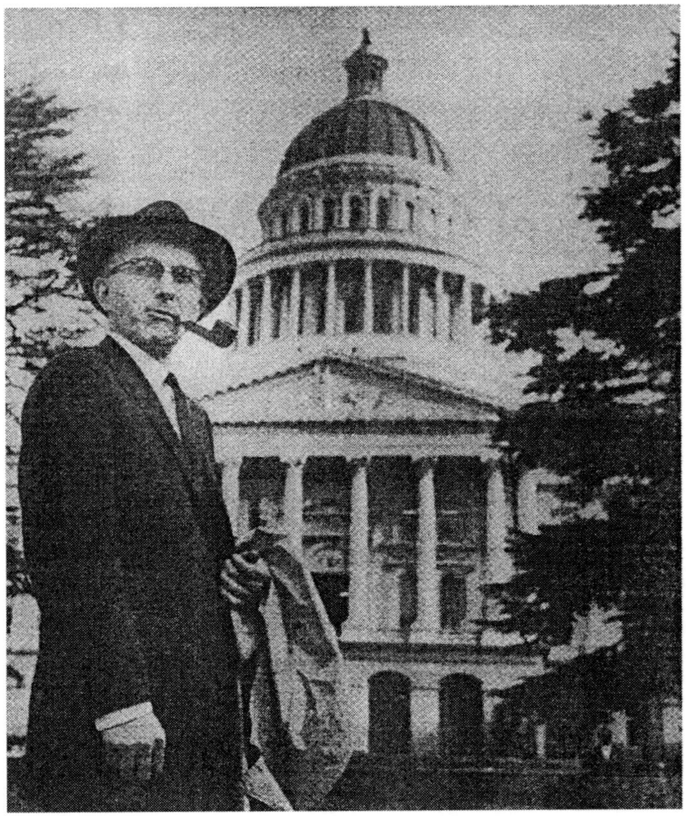

Sydney, the journalist

Even Richard Nixon once tried to get Sydney fired. When Nixon was running for governor, Sydney accused him of not understanding state problems and trying to use the governorship as a springboard to the presidency. "No [California politician] had a longer career as a smear artist than Richard Nixon... He gave dirty politics a bad name," he wrote. An angry Nixon sent some of his men to pressure Sydney's boss, who said, "I'll decide who gets hired and fired on this paper." He then "showed the thugs the door."

I glanced at this man who had been

For Sydney, his allegiance was always to the people of his country, always making sure they got the whole truth. He wasn't a man to mince words when confronted with powerful politicians.

called the "Dean of Northern California Political Writers" by former San Francisco mayor Willie Brown; served as president of the San Francisco Press Club; received prestigious awards from the Associated Press and Librarians' Association of America; ridden on Air Force One and attended political conventions; interviewed David Ben Gurion, Ronald Reagan, Pat Brown, George Christopher, Earl Warren, Lyndon B. Johnson and Jimmy Carter. And what I wanted to ask him was how it felt to be here in his room, now, reliving his memories—alone.

But Sydney kept talking, explaining how he had a White House press pass and participated in White House press corps meetings with President Johnson. The first time he met with Johnson, Sydney realized that he had just been "let into the office of the most powerful man in the world." And all Sydney, a true American journalist, could think was hope to God he doesn't blow it.

Then there was his famous scoop of the AP wire. While entering the capitol building in Sacramento, Sydney heard shots across the lawn. He ran towards the pay phones in the Senator Hotel, where he had spent many nights and interviewed famous people, and called his office. "There was an assassination attempt on Gerald Ford!" Sydney said, breathing heavily as he remembered how the secret service agents had saved the President. The city desk explained that the wires hadn't picked it up yet, and Sydney replied, "No, I am ahead of those guys! I was there! I saw a woman attempt to assassinate President Ford!" He had scooped the wires on the attempted assassination—a feat that wasn't an easy one.

For Sydney, his allegiance was always to the people of his country, always making sure they got the whole truth. He wasn't a man to mince words when confronted with powerful politicians. Instead he confronted them with their mistakes, saying that Ronald Reagan "seemed to live in the past... He presumably knows, though, that neither California nor the nation can go back to how it used to be." Or he called his readers to action by asking, "Where have the issue fighters gone? Where are the candidates who deal with subjects that matter?"

But none of that would compare to his proudest working moment. He had been selected by the Jewish Labor Delegation to tour Israel. Jeanette joined him. They visited the Dead Sea, Masada, Tel Aviv, Jerusalem, the Wailing Wall, and when they arrived at the Sea of Galilee—a place he had read about his whole life—he had the opportunity to meet the George Washington of Israel: David Ben Gurion. The famous statesman was well into retirement by then. He had bodyguards and doctors surrounding him as Sydney approached their meeting place on a balcony overlooking the wide blue sea. The first thing Sydney noticed about this great leader was his "trademark shock of white hair." Trying to hide his excitement, Sydney asked about the prospects for peace in Israel. Ben Gurion was confident that eventually the Israelis would make peace with the Arabs.

"This was someone I had read about, seen in pictures. He did amazing things in establishing the state of Israel. I was proud to sit with him. Proud of myself for having come that far," recalled Sydney. His description of this moment made me realize that Sydney, too, was a legend—a man from another time who fought for this country, who believed in the innate goodness of the United States, regardless of our current politics; a man who helped make or break presidents and senators, governors and mayors; and a man who, steeped in knowledge of the past, was optimistic about the future. It was an optimism few in my generation felt during this upcoming Presidential election of 2004.

It was the preservation of his religion that forced his family out of Russia, that carried them safely to the United States, that harbored them against the cruelty of others, that brought them closer to their neighbors.

The next Wednesday was Rosh Hashanah, the Jewish New Year. Sydney excitedly explained that his Jewish identity had always been a huge part of his existence. It was the lifeline that helped him get through. His faith was intense, unshakeable, immoveable, true. He was born with it, raised with it, believed in it. It was the preservation of his religion that forced his family out of Russia, that carried them safely to the United States, that harbored them against the cruelty of others, that brought them closer to their neighbors. It was the reason he fought for his country, lost his hearing and later his vision. It was what created the bond between him and Jeanette, his love for his parents, and his pride in being successful as a Jewish writer. It was everything.

Rosh Hashanah took him back to his childhood. For the big holiday, he got to stay out of school. It represented growing up, another year, a new beginning. He got to wear a suit. It was not like a calendar New Year with cocktail parties and friends. For Rosh Hashanah, people prayed. They collected at his mother's house, cleaned thoroughly and then prepared a feast. The evening would culminate a day of synagogue, where the rabbi would blow the lamb's horn to signify the start of a new year. And when they returned home, his mother would cover her head with a white cloth and sing her prayers. Then the whole family would gather around the dinner table to share sweet wine, challah, brisket, potatoes, rugaleh and other sweets. The festivities would end with the women clearing the plates and retreating to the kitchen to share stories, while the men would convene outside to smoke pipes and talk about current events. Each year, Sydney the child, craved for the time when he would belong to that group of men sharing grown-up ideas outside in the late summer heat.

Today, Sydney's family would come to share the holiday services with him at Reutlinger. His son and daughter-in-law would drive in from Clear Lake, pick up Jeanette, and arrive for synagogue just after dinner. Sydney hoped to get called to the Torah that evening, even though he could not see to read anymore. The rabbi would help him, like she did the other vision-impaired residents. It was possible that his son, Michael, would be called too. It would please Sydney to stand before the congregation with his son. It was an honor like no other. Tonight, Sydney would pray for forgiveness for whatever he has done wrong that year and under his God, he would be forgiven. "I have done as best as I could. Now, I am just glad to still be alive."

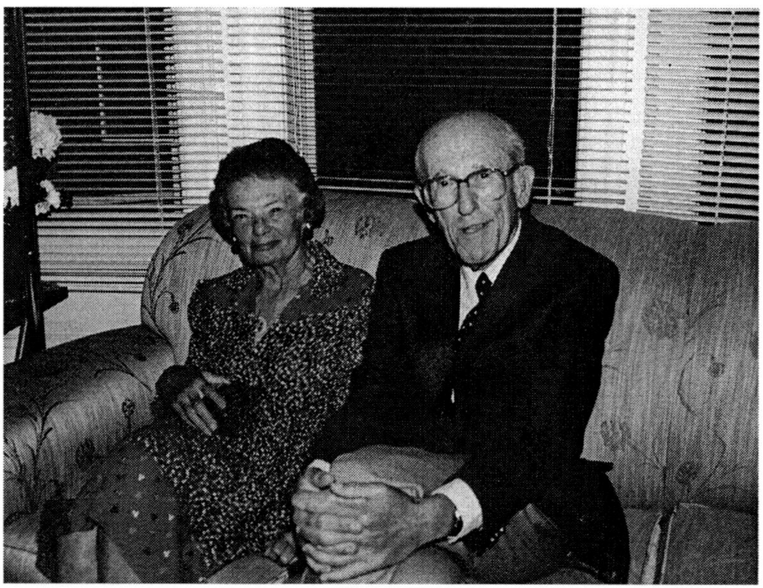

Sydney and his wife Jeanette

It would be two months before I would visit Sydney again. I, like the rest of San Francisco and the country, would be wrapped up in the presidential election. And the day after the results would kamikaze their way into the lives of the American people, I would return to the only person I knew who could make any sense of the state of American politics.

There he was, lying on the bed, with his arms encircling his adoring wife. The two of them huddled together like survivors, clinging to the breath of the other, letting their embrace act as a catalyst for communication. Being away from his wife was difficult. After sixty-one years of marriage, so many of them apart, just like now when they saw each other but once a week, here were Sydney and Jeanette on this bed, still able to show each other love.

I told them not to get up, apologized for interrupting the precious few moments they would have together and then said I just had one question today: "What now?"

He smiled, patted my hand, then said, "It will all be okay."

And there I was, another person struck by the optimism of Sydney Kossen. It was the same kind of optimism that Sydney had heard from David Ben Gurion. I understood why his wife stayed with him over the five years of being separated by the war. She had endured the later years, when he traveled so often for work and only occasionally made it home for dinner. His touch infected me with his confidence. It invoked me not to worry about another four years of oppressive government, strife in the Middle East, wars—just focus on the good, just have faith, and remember who and what you love.

[Sydney's touch] invoked me not to worry about another four years of oppressive government, strife in the Middle East, wars—just focus on the good, just have faith, and remember who and what you love.

I returned around Hanukkah for my last interview. When I entered his room, Sydney hugged me as though I were family and began to explain how he retired from the *Examiner* around the time his grandchildren were born. It would be this way with Sydney, this mambo between work and family. How he would not be home much to see the events of his children and grandchildren's lives, yet would claim their graduations and births as the delights of his existence.

Those significant family milestones, and his later work.

After retirement, Sydney wrote articles for the *Washington Post* Sunday section and *Harpers*. It was for these articles that he was honored and would later win awards and plaques. His last job was volunteering for Dianne Feinstein's mayoral campaign. What made him proudest in his service was not the fact that his wife had been the mayor's Sunday school teacher, but that Mayor Feinstein had remembered Jeanette Kossen's delicate good looks and impenetrable charms. Sydney was Mayor Feinstein's press secretary, proud to be of service to the "first Jewish mayor of San Francisco since Adolf Sutro."

Then Sydney had an accident. Listening to an audio book as he walked to get the mail, Sydney tripped and fell. He fractured his skull, releasing blood onto his brain. Ever since then, he has needed a walker and constant care. He went to three different centers before finding his present "home" at

Reutlinger—an oasis of Jewish tradition. Here he could eat Kosher food, attend synagogue once a week, pray with others, speak Yiddish, all in a safe, loving atmosphere. This was the way Jeanette and Sydney agreed to handle these winter years. "Now, I am in the infirmities of old age," Sydney said, "I accept it. Adjust to it the best I can. I am like my mother. I have a card-file memory. Memories become dim, just like my vision. "

"I am like my mother. I have a card-file memory. Memories become dim, just like my vision."

I felt him slipping into exhaustion and tried to steer him back to more energizing topics by asking, "What is something you still wish to do?"

Sydney explained that he wished he had written a book about American politics. He also wished that he had taken his son fishing under the Golden Gate Bridge. His one hobby was fishing, a reminder of his years at sea. He would bob under the bridge, letting the fog take him back to the days when the land seemed to stop existing. He never took his son, because he was afraid Michael would get "as sick as the Filipino monkey" that his Navy crew had adopted as a mascot.

"But, really, there are no deep sorrows," Sydney relented. "I am happy. I got to cover presidential campaigns; got to speak to some great men."

I then asked him about the joys of being eighty-eight.

Sydney laughed. "If you live to be eighty-eight," he reached over and touched my arm, "well, you'll have friends, I hope. And you'll be happy among them. There is joy in looking back, yes. I accept that this is the way it is."

I suddenly grasped why I needed to be a part of this project and why we all need to reminisce with our elders. As a young progressive person, I constantly looked to the future to change, to evolve. Yet here was a man who had only the past left to guide him forward. His life passed so swiftly and here he was now, surrounded by a Jewish atmosphere, with his memories, his occasional stolen moments with his wife, wheelchair rides with Michael, conversations with residents, rabbis, nurses and doctors, but his lifeline existed in the past. And that was what made Sydney so wise. No longer did he rush forward to the next moment. Instead he calmly meditated upon what has passed, what lives in the years gone by, understanding that in the end it will be only the memories that calm and comfort us. ■

WRITER'S PROFILE

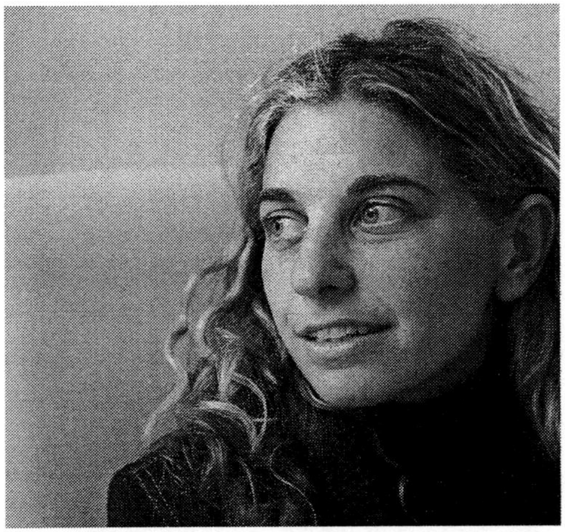

Michele Bigley

I started writing so that I could tell the stories of the amazing people I meet. Sydney Kossen is one of them. It was my honor to learn from and share in his experiences.

It was also my honor to chronicle the lives of my family's elders in a very personal way. I interviewed my grandmothers soon after each was diagnosed with terminal cancer, and wrote their life stories for their offspring.

On a professional note, I am a writer and educator, with an MFA from Antioch College. I teach creative writing to little tykes in the Mission district of San Francisco and composition at Foothill College, a community college in Los Altos. I recently finished a novel entitled "Where the Ten Meets the One" and am beginning a new novel. My fiction, poetry, and nonfiction have appeared in *Tea Party, Moxie, Storyglossia,* and *Coloring Book: An Anthology of Multicultural Writers.*

JOE MORENO

Mountain View Healthcare Center
Mountain View, California
with
Rebekah Eppley

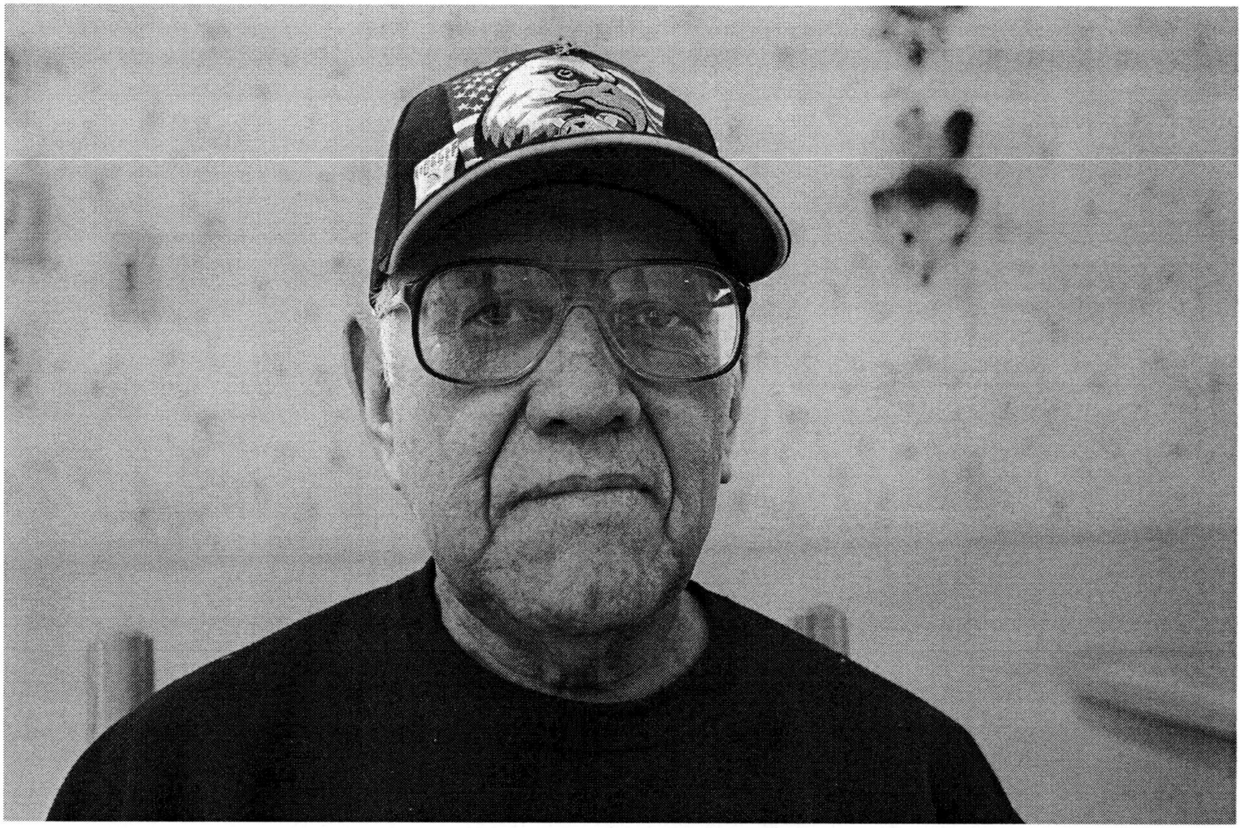

"We take care of each other"

"Who is Joe Moreno?" I'm thinking as I make my first trip to the nursing home. I haven't prepared any real questions for our initial meeting, thinking it best to simply talk freely and get to know each other a bit before we launch into his history. I wonder if Joe will remind me of someone, or if we will feel unfamiliar to each other. And how will he feel about his current living situation? Will our meeting be awkward, with long gaps of silence or will he be a talker? And how much will he be willing to share with me, a complete stranger? So many questions pass through my mind. By the time I reach the nursing home, I feel anxious and almost dread walking through the front doors.

"I always knew how to work," he tells me. "And I've never stopped. I'm still working, even now."

My mood quickly shifts as I enter the dining room: a bright, colorful space at Mountain View Healthcare Center. It's a room that could easily be part of a family home. Wallpaper of yellow flowers on a white background covers the walls. The curtained window on the back wall overlooks plants and shrubbery. An old-fashioned popcorn maker is tucked in the corner near the window, and three wooden tables stand along the walls, their ladder-back chairs in rows against the side of the room. White and yellow tiles stretch across the floor, still damp from a recent mopping. There is an order to this room, Joe will later explain—a purpose to the setup.

Joe sits at the head of the table next to the window and motions for me to sit in the chair on his right that he's pulled over for my visit. He's wearing a black sweatshirt with the sleeves bunched up a bit between his wrist and elbow and a baseball cap with an eagle emblem and an American flag pinned to the front. The cap, I soon learn, is part of his regular attire. Inside his left wrist I notice a black and red heart tattoo, matched by another on top of his left hand. A black target is tattooed on the flesh just above the wrist inside his right arm.

At first Joe seems a bit stern. He shakes my hand and quickly launches into a discussion about work. "I always knew how to work," he tells me. "And I've never stopped. I'm still working, even now." Shifting into an explanation of his present "job," he describes how he prepares the dining room where we sit by moving the chairs to the corner and along the walls to make room for the wheelchair-bound residents. As he speaks, he illustrates and motions with his hands, showing me where things go and how they're done.

"See, we put those chairs over there next to the wall, so when they

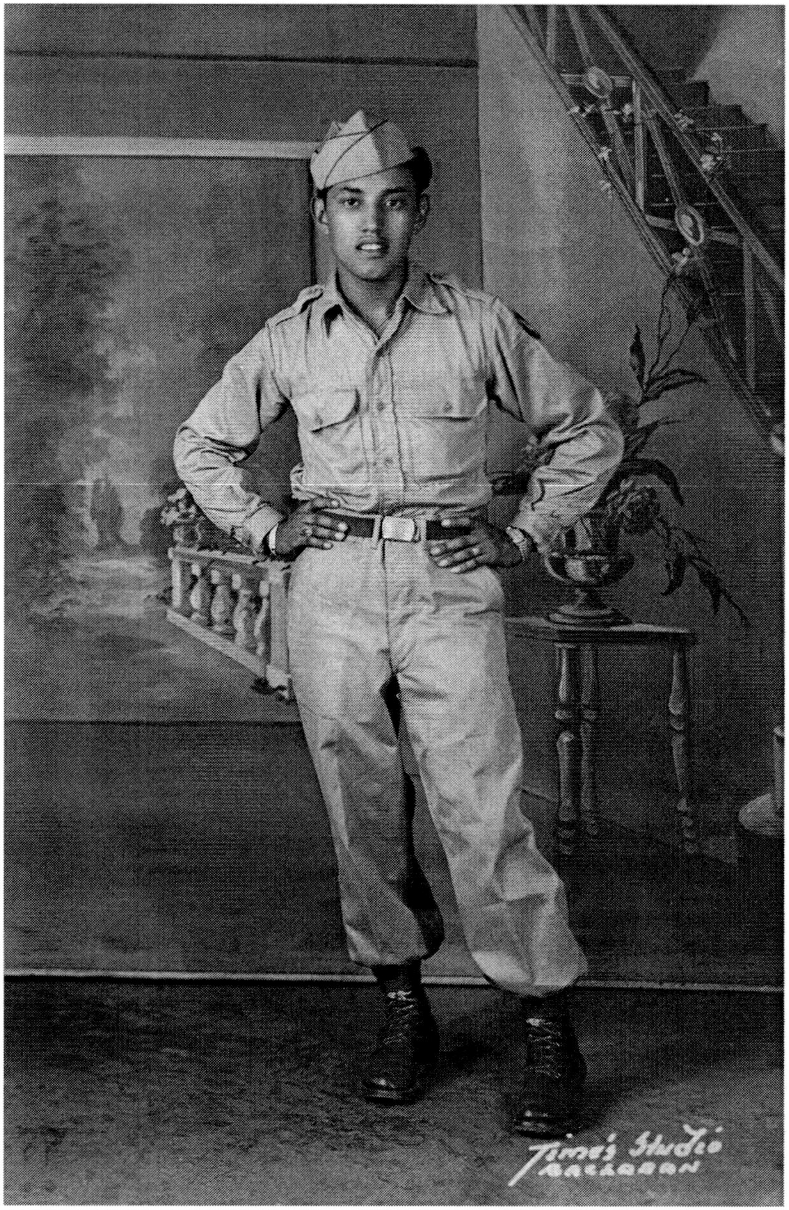

Joe in his Air Force uniform

wheel people in there's a place for them to sit at the tables. We all have our place." He motions to the table across the room and tells me that's where he sits.

After mealtimes, the floors are swept and mopped. While Joe doesn't perform this particular duty, he shows me, with much precision, how this is done, illustrating the exact way to hold the mop.

Sometime during that first encounter, Joe flashes a quick smile and I sense a warmth in him. That smile alone is enough to make me want to return. I realize, as I leave that afternoon, that Joe's voice has already filled my head—the lilting tone as he sounds out the o's or emphasizes a word is like music. The cadence and rhythm of his language remain with me long after I leave.

Sometime during that first encounter, Joe flashes a quick smile and I sense a warmth in him. That smile alone is enough to make me want to return.

Joe is alert and engaged and, from what I can tell, moves with relative ease. I'm not sure why he's living in the home. I understand, from our brief conversation, that he came for care after a back injury from which he seems to have recovered. And yet he remains.

When I return the following Saturday, I find Joe in his bedroom, which he shares with two other residents. Joe's bed is in the middle, separated from the other two men by privacy curtains. Each man has a nightstand, dresser, television set and some personal belongings. An orange and black Giants blanket covers Joe's bed. A strand of Mardi Gras beads hangs from the wall over his pillow. "I won those at Bingo," he tells me. "We play Bingo every Saturday. We all love it 'cause we act like kids. Everyone wants to win something."

Across the room, a 5 by 7 photo of a young Joe dressed in his Air Force uniform shares space with a 49ers roster on the wall. Beneath his television set are photos of family and friends. He points out his daughter, Teresa, and her three children Selica, Derek and Requel and Selica's children, Joe's great-grandchildren, Isaac and Yamila.

"They all came to visit me the other day. It was lunchtime and I looked up and there was my daughter, her married daughter and her two kids standing in the doorway. My granddaughter has a little one like that," he holds his hand just above his knee to illustrate the size of his great-granddaughter. "Everyone was looking at me and I said, 'That's my family!'" Joe breaks into a

"I never knew there were places like this," he tells me. "I told my daughter I'm not getting out of here. She said I could live with her, but I like it here. This is a beautiful place."

smile and shakes his head as if he can't believe his good fortune.

"My daughter told the little one to go to grandpa and she walked right up to me. That's my great-granddaughter. Last time I saw her she was a baby, but when you see them walking it's different. She came right up to me and knew who I was. I'll remember that for a long time."

Joe reaches for a walker next to his dresser and pulls it toward him. "I have to use this or they scold me," he laughs. Pointing to the dining room across the hall he says, "Let's go."

Inside the dining room Joe motions for me to sit at the table along the left wall and he takes a seat at the head of the table, establishing our seating arrangement for the remainder of our meetings. "This is where I sit every day," he explains. "And grandma, she sits over there." He points to the chair to his left. "She's ninety something years old and very sharp. And she always sits next to me. So I talk to her. Everyone talks to each other. We're like a family."

Joe begins most of our sessions in this manner, telling me a bit about the residents at the home and how he's spent the past several days. I'm interested in this aspect of his life – how he's come to make the nursing home his permanent home and why he's remained.

I ask Joe if he enjoys living here. He emphatically tells me, "Oh yeah, yeah. It's nice. Real nice. And I try to do what I can to help them out here. I don't have to do it, but I like to help out. And they appreciate that. They don't try to keep you prisoner. You've seen movies about that, but not here. They're beautiful here."

I quickly learn that Joe injured his back at his last job at Mountain View Community Center, where he worked stocking shelves and distributing food to area residents in need. "I always gave them [recipients of the food] a little extra," he tells me. "If we were supposed to give them two of something, I'd give them four."

He doesn't remember coming to Mountain View Healthcare Center because he was in excruciating pain. That was nearly a year ago and he's been living here ever since, after his doctor told him he would no longer be able to live alone.

"I never knew there were places like this," he tells me. "I told my daughter I'm not getting out of here. She said I could live with her, but I like it here. This is a beautiful place. We take care of each other. They brought a lady today. Right away she liked it because everyone welcomed her. We tell her this is our home, we're together and we'll be with you. And that's what it takes. I've seen it with my own eyes." Joe emphasizes this last point by firmly placing his clenched fist on the table, and then continues.

"The ones that are helping out, we know what the others like. We don't push them fast in their wheelchairs, but slowly, like they were your mother or something. The last time a new lady came she was kind of scared. I said, 'Don't worry. Nobody's gonna hurt you.' I tell her, 'If anyone hurts you I'll ...'" Joe forces a scowl, then punches his hand into his fist, laughing.

Although I don't know it yet, this early visit captures the essence of Joe in his earlier life. As our meetings continue, I'll often catch glimpses of the young, first-generation Mexican man who began his working life as a child in the fields between California's Imperial Valley and San Jose and who was fiercely protective of his friends, family and home.

"They just jumped the fence at Mexicali," Joe tells me when I ask how his parents crossed the border. "Everyone did it like that back then."

Jose Moreno was born in Brawley, a town in Southern California's Imperial Valley, on February 2, 1928. "Groundhog's Day," he tells me laughing. "I know the groundhog pretty well." He was named for his father, a Mexican immigrant originally from Durango.

"A lot of Mexican families call their sons 'junior' after their father," Joe tells me. They'll call you 'junior, junior.'" Joe repeats the words in a taunting voice to show disgust. "I didn't like that so they gave me a nickname. Pepe. Everybody in my family called me Pepe. They didn't call me Joe or nothing. When I went to school, I had to learn English then and that's when they started calling me Joe. But all my friends called me Pepe."

While working on a ranch in Durango, Joe's father, Joe Sr., met and fell in love with his future wife, Anita, the rancher's daughter. He was eventually fired when Anita's father learned of their attraction to one another. Work was scarce so Joe's parents came to the United States, where they married and raised a family. They arrived in Brawley, California as a young couple in the 1920s.

"They just jumped the fence at Mexicali," Joe tells me when I ask how his parents crossed the border. "Everyone did it like that back then. They didn't have problems because there was always work to be done in the fields. They needed people to work and we knew how to work."

When I ask if he still has family in Durango, Joe tells me, "no," then thinks for a few minutes and reconsiders. "Probably. But I don't know anything about that. When my parents came here they never looked back."

As far as Joe remembers, his parents never told stories about their life in Mexico. He learned the story of his parent's meeting and subsequent journey to the United States from his oldest sister, Anita, named for her mother.

"Working just comes naturally to me."

Joe's mother died when he was young, but he hasn't forgotten her. "I barely knew her. I was small, but I remember her. I don't remember how she died. It was from a disease. Maybe cancer. I don't remember, just that she died in her sleep. But I remember her," he assures me.

After his mother died, Anita took over as caregiver for her siblings, John, Frank, Joe, and Nelly. Another brother, Felix, died before Joe was born. He doesn't know much about Felix or how he died, but Joe makes sure to include him when he speaks of his brothers and sisters.

Reflecting on those years after his mother died, Joe remembers Anita as having a hard hand, but taking good care of the family. He and his siblings had already started working in the fields during those early years, when they were still children. Back then the work felt more like play to Joe. The adults gave him a bucket and told him to pick what he could. He explains that the children would pull fruit from the lower branches of the trees that they could reach and eventually learned to pick from the higher branches by watching the adults.

"I learned real quick. By the time I was about thirteen I was working for real. There's a right way to do it. If you don't learn it the right way, it's like pushing through a wall, but if you learn to do it the right way you go through the wall. Like here. It's easy for me to work here because I know how to do it. I know how to set things up to help out. Working just comes naturally to me."

The family would come from Brawley up to San Jose for work in the summers where they'd pick cherries, pears, peaches and muscatel grapes. Joe explains that the grapes were the easiest crop for him to pick because they were so big and came in fat bunches. Peaches ranked low on his list because the fuzz rubbed off on his hands and arms and left his skin itchy all day.

Joe remembers picking plums, grapes and tomatoes as a child. Back then Mountain View was a small, agricultural town consisting mainly of orchards. "It was nothing like this now," he tells me. The main street right here was Castro. And later on there was a post office. And further down there was movies. And it was all one street and everything else was orchards."

Joe, his siblings and father would live in a cabin or small house provided by the farmer. On Saturday or Sunday they'd go shopping with the money they made during the week.

"And then, every year after we finished our work, one of the neighbors might need help, so he'd ask the farmers if he could lend his people. That's how they'd help each other. So then we'd go and pick the neighbors' crops. And every year we'd come to the same rancher. He had good neighbors and would lend us to them. So we used to go back with lots of money," he laughs.

"My dad was real polite. And he always tried to help somebody."

During the winters in Brawley, Joe's father sometimes worked as a carpenter or a cook, supporting Joe and his siblings. Joe speaks fondly of his father and attributes his work ethic and manners to him:

"My dad was real polite. And he always tried to help somebody. They'd call him Mr. Moreno because he would help people with money and he was a carpenter and would always help out. He knew everything. If people asked him to help build houses he would do it. And he was a plumber, too. Everything, everything. He could do everything."

"And he taught you?" I ask.

"Yeah and my brother John—he was the oldest in our family. He was like a father to me. He didn't call me 'Pepe,' he called me 'my son.' He was a real good worker. And I never heard him say a bad word about anyone, I swear to God. He was a real good man and he worked hard. Just like me. I'm still working." Joe then quickly changes the subject, as he takes on his role of "guide" at the care center. "Did I show you that other room, where they have the activities?"

I shake my head no. Already Joe is in a standing position and reaching for his walker. "Come on, I'll take you."

I follow Joe down the hallway to the activities room, where he pushes the door open and waits for me to enter. The room feels open and airy. Sliding glass doors look onto a back patio. A paperback-filled bookcase stretches along the right wall. On the wall opposite the bookcase is a long cabinet with drawers and cupboards. A piano stands at the back of the room, next to the glass doors and a whiteboard announcing the day's activities, morning Tai Chi and bingo at 2:00. Running down the center of the room and off to the left side are two long dining tables.

Joe opens a cabinet drawer and shows me the tablecloths he spreads

"I thought when I came here it would be like, you just stay in bed, but no, they always got something for us to do. We've got bingo and movies and we even had a Superbowl party."

over the table each morning in preparation for breakfast. A woman pushes open the door and says hello. "That's my boss, Mary," Joe tells me. "She's a beautiful person. She and A.J. are the ones who set up the activities. They're both real beautiful people. I thought when I came here it would be like, you just stay in bed, but no, they always got something for us to do. We've got bingo and movies and we even had a Superbowl party."

Joe tells me that he'd lived with his daughter for a brief time before he was injured, while recovering from pneumonia. She'd offered her home to him again after his injury, but he prefers the nursing home. His daughter's home is in Pleasanton, at least thirty miles from Mountain View and far from all that is familiar to him. At the home, he has friends and community.

As we walk back down the hallway, Joe points out a large calendar listing events for the month. I quickly read through the upcoming events – Art Appreciation, Monday Matinee and Popcorn, Bingo, Gospel Hour, Daily News, Trivia, Candlelight Dinner, Poetry Hour and Armchair Travel are just a few. "The days go by real quick," Joe tells me. "'Cause there's always something for me to do."

During another visit I catch Joe just as he's headed down the hallway for his twice-daily walk around the home.

"Did you forget I was coming?"

"No, no. I remembered." Then he laughs. "I remembered when I saw you."

Every day Joe makes his rounds, visiting his friends down the hall and in the neighboring wing of the home. Sometimes he'll pass an elder struggling with her wheelchair and he'll give her a push to help her along. "They know it's me and they smile. It reminds me of when I used to stop to help someone along the side of a road with a flat tire, except now it's a wheelchair I'm helping with," Joe laughs.

As we settle into our places in the dining room, Joe tells me that he's forgotten some things, like dates and the names of places, or the order of things. "It was a long time ago," he says. But he always remembers the details of his work and the times he shared with family and friends.

The names of friends are easily recalled, like Manuel Mendez from Long Beach, whom Joe met when he was drafted at the end of World War II. The two met at a camp for recruits and were stationed together throughout their time in the service. Many of the new recruits were separated after training, so Joe feels lucky that he and his new *compadre* were able to stay together and were eventually stationed in the same barracks.

Joe was sent to the Philippines with the Air Force after the war, on a peace mission, he says, to help clean up.

"My brother, Frank, he was there during the fighting and he saw some terrible things. He did the hard part. He went all the way to Germany and when he came back he'd have terrible nightmares. He wouldn't talk to anybody about this except his wife. Well, you know what they say, 'War is hell.' And they're right."

"And in the hill you could see planes in the side where they crashed. It was terrible. I saw a lot of stuff and I couldn't believe it."

As Joe tells the story he remembers that an entertainer was at the home the previous week. During his performance, he asked if any of the female residents worked as riveters during the war. Joe was surprised when three of his friends raised their hands in response. He's delighted as he shares this information with me, having discovered something new about his friends.

Later the performer asked how many men had served in World War II. An older man sitting next to Joe revealed that he'd been a bombardier. Joe recounts an exchange between him and the former bombardier:

"He looked at me and said, 'How about you son, did you serve in the war?' I said, 'Yeah, but I served when the war was over' and he said, 'But you served' and he shook my hand and I felt real good and I told him, 'No, I should be shaking your hand because *you* did the hard job.' And he almost cried."

Although the war was over when Joe served, the sad remnants of the disaster remained. Joe talks about arriving in the port of Manila after a week aboard ship:

"You'd see sunk ships. You'd have to go real slow because all through the bay these ships were sunk upright. And in the hill you could see planes in the side where they crashed. It was terrible. I saw a lot of stuff and I couldn't believe it. We saw a lot of the barracks that were all shot up. And the officer's quarters. Everything was shattered."

Local people, including children, walked the streets with machine guns in the scene Joe describes. He seems incredulous, even as he recounts the experience fifty years later. "I'd seen movies," he tells me. "But nothing like that in real life."

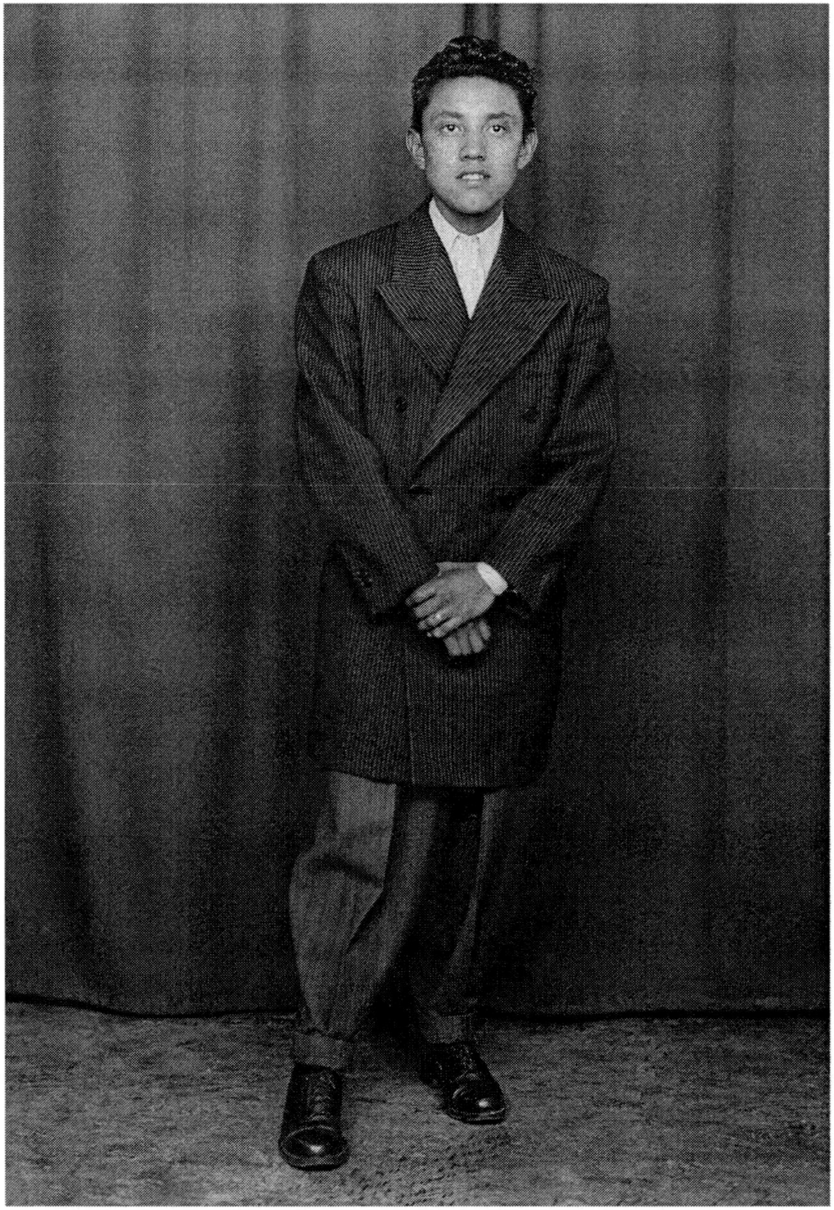

Joe in his zoot suit

During his duty in the Philippines, Joe endured the racial prejudice of the other soldiers and talks about how others in the barracks often urged the two Latinos—Joe and Manuel—to box for entertainment.

"A lot of nights they had boxing and they all wanted us to fight because we were the same size, but I didn't want to and he didn't want to because, you know, when you fight he'd punch you hard and I'd punch him and you'd get mad and we said 'No, our friendship is friendship and no fighting.' But they wanted us to fight because we were the same size; we were Mexicans. I had a few fights there and I showed them what I could do, you know, I could fight dirty or clean or whatever. There was a lot of prejudice in the military. They'd call me a dirty Mexican. I didn't say nothing at first. I didn't know the score, and then I decided I wasn't going to take it. I learned to defend myself when I was young. In my hometown, you gotta learn not to back up."

"There was a lot of prejudice in the military. They'd call me a dirty Mexican."

"Why was that?"

"Well, it's a tradition over there, you know. You don't back up from nobody even if he hits you, and then other people will respect you, and then nobody will pick on you. But I had a lot of friends," Joe assures me. "We had about forty of us in the gang."

"Was that when you were growing up?"

"No, we were already grown up. We were about sixteen or seventeen. But we didn't do nothing bad."

Joe makes it clear that his gang wasn't like today's gangs. "It wasn't even really a gang. Sort of a gang, but we had a good time. We played sports together a lot. Speedball and basketball. We were never in fights. Well, when somebody came to our neighborhood and tried to get tough, but we had a good time, too."

"So the gang was started to protect each other?"

"Yeah, to protect each other and the neighborhood. We had this one guy, Gilbert Lopez. He had hands like a baseball mitt. If he hit you one time, you'd be out. Big hands," Joe stretches the words for emphasis. "Every Saturday and Sunday guys from the other towns would try to come over here and go to our dances, but you weren't supposed to go to each other's towns."

Dancing was a big part of Joe's life in both Brawley and in San Jose. When he lived in Southern California he used to cross over the border into Mexicali, a twenty-two mile drive from Brawley, to go dancing with his friends from the gang.

There wasn't a drinking age in Mexicali so Joe and his buddies frequented what he describes as a type of drive-in bar where they could order anything they wanted before making their way to the dances. It was during a trip to Mexicali that Joe and his friends decided on a name for their gang.

"We got to talking because we'd all been together since we were kids and we were in a gang, but we didn't have a name. So we started talking about it and then we got the cigarette lighter from the car and shhhh, like that," Joe presses an imaginary lighter into his inner left hand. The lighter made a target imprint into the flesh of their hands, which is how they decided to name themselves the Targets.

"And then we gave ourselves tattoos. My friend did this one," he tells me pointing to his right hand, "because I couldn't do it left-handed. It hurt, but I had to finish it. Everyone in my town had a tattoo. I always had a lot of friends, like this one here," Joe tells me, suddenly thrust back to the present.

A woman with smiling eyes wheels herself up to the table. "That's grandma," explains Joe. "Remember I told you about her?" She introduces herself to me as Velma.

"She's waiting for bingo," Joe adds. "And I'm gonna walk all over them today," Velma retorts. We all share a laugh before she wheels herself back out the door.

After just two weeks of visits, Joe announced that he didn't have anything else to tell me. He'd told it all, he said, and seemed frustrated that he didn't have anything else to share. He had already generously shared many stories about his work and family, but I felt like there was still so much more to know. He agreed to see me one more time, but insisted there was nothing more to tell.

I remember feeling worried that perhaps he was uncomfortable with me or with the project. Was I bringing up painful memories? Or was I interrupting his busy schedule? He always seemed on his way to something else when I arrived, after all, and already I sensed that he had a rich life at the home.

Maybe he had enough people to talk to. I'd hoped this wasn't the case. I so much enjoyed meeting with Joe and hearing his stories and I didn't want our time to end so quickly. Already I'd grown accustomed to the intonations in his voice and the sound of his laughter that seemed to come to him so easily.

After what was to be our final meeting, Joe seemed more relaxed and told me he enjoyed talking with me and he was remembering things he hadn't thought about in a long time. When I asked him if bringing up those memories was upsetting, he assured me that it wasn't. I felt like Joe was offering me a gift in agreeing to continue our meetings.

Now, after our weekly meetings, I leave with such vivid images of both Joe's earlier life and his current life. I feel haunted by his description of the Philippines post- World War II and feel his excitement when he tells me about a fiddler who performed one afternoon at the home. "Oh, how he made that fiddle cry," he tells me.

I sense Joe's tenderness when he describes the importance of his friends in both his past and his current life in the nursing home. And when he takes me back to his early years with the gang, I can't help but feel a sense of melancholy, since I know he's lost touch with all those old friends.

Sometimes I think back to that first meeting when I wondered, "Who is Joe?" Now, it feels like ages ago, even though I've only known him for several months. I realize there will be many things I'll never know about my new friend and how limited I'll be in trying to tell his story. I want to remain true to that story, to capture Joe's experience and yet it comes to me second-hand, after decades that have altered his memory. It comes filtered, too, through me and my experience of Joe.

I want to remain true to that story, to capture Joe's experience and yet it comes to me second-hand, after decades that have altered his memory.

And yet I feel I am beginning to know Joe gradually through bits and pieces of his stories. When I see the tattoo on his hands, I imagine him in a car with his old friends, driving across the Mexican border, excited about a night on the town. When I look at the picture of the young man dressed in uniform hanging on his wall, I see a bit of what Joe saw as he sailed into Manila fifty years ago. And always I'm ready for more stories.

The time Joe spent in the Philippines was the longest period that he'd been separated from his family. He recalls, with much sadness, an incident that occurred back home while he was away.

His youngest sister, Nelly, and Joe's two young nephews were walking home from school together when they came upon an old storage shed. Curious, like all kids, they went inside to explore and discovered a box of discarded dynamite caps. Unaware of what they were, they began throwing the caps back and forth between them. When one of the children missed "the catch," a cap hit the ground and exploded, killing Joe's nephew, George, and blinding both Nelly and her cousin, Arthur.

"It was real sad. Because they were just little kids. I could've come home for the funeral," Joe says with a tone of regret, "but I found out too late." He goes on to describe how the surviving children "were real low, real depressed because they thought their life was over and I guess we did too." They later went a school for the blind and learned Braille. But the story brightens. "Later Nelly met a white boy there. Russell. He's real big," Joe emphasizes his size, laughing. "He's not short like me. And they got married and have a girl and a boy. They're big kids like their father. Real nice kids. Big. They live in Gilroy now. They're a real nice family."

"And you know, I always tried to treat everyone the same because you never know when things can change. When something might happen, even in your own family, even now. You've gotta treat everyone with respect."

Joe ends the story with a moral, stating what I realize is one of the guiding principles of his life: "And you know, I always tried to treat everyone the same because you never know when things can change. When something might happen, even in your own family, even now. You've gotta treat everyone with respect. I've always tried to treat everyone the same, even here."

Rainy weather has transformed my usual forty-five minute drive to Mountain View to an hour's trip, but I find Joe this Saturday morning patiently waiting for me in his room, the newspaper spread open in front of him on the bed. "I read the paper every day," Joe announces.

I'm wondering where our conversation will take us today. So often when we meet we take a circuitous route. I'll think we're talking about one thing only to discover that the conversation has shifted and we've landed on another path. At first, the detours and side conversations frustrated me because I felt like I wasn't keeping our conversation on track, but I've come to accept the meandering of our discussion, realizing that it best represents the movement of Joe's life, traveling back and forth between north and south. It's also more true to the way memory actually works. I'm enjoying learning about Joe in the way his memory dictates, rather than following a linear path that I might try to dictate through my questions.

Today, it's his newspaper reading that sets the topic of our conversation. "There was an article about Alum Rock Park the other day and when I saw that, it brought back lots of memories," Joe tells me as we pull our chairs up to the dining room table.

Joe and his family often spent Sunday afternoons at the park nestled in the hills of San Jose. "We used to go on picnics and swim. When my daughter was small I'd take her swimming."

Joe is an excellent swimmer and diver—a skill he learned in the irrigation canals during his early years in Brawley. But his dream to swim on the high school swim team was never realized, he tells me emphatically. Though he made the swim team, he left school after just a year, feeling like he was never given a real chance to succeed. The racism of the small southern California town where he was raised got in the way.

"I wanted to swim so bad, but there was prejudice. It was a white world. They were nasty so finally I quit. We used to go to the canals where I lived and I'd beat anyone at swimming. And diving." Joe talks about how his mother went swimming with him, and how they had "a beautiful car. I even had a '51 Chevy. I always made good money. I had good jobs. I wanted to stay in high school, but there was real prejudice. 'Mexican greasers' they called us and I couldn't stand it."

Joe draws an imaginary map on the table to show how the town was segregated. "We lived here," he says, pointing to the spot where his neighborhood would be. "And the tracks are here. And the white people would say, 'Get back on the other side of the tracks.'" Later, after the war, he explained, each side of town had its own movie house. "We [the Mexicans] had our own [theater], but there were good American movies in their theater. We had Mexican movies. We wanted to see the American movies, but they said 'You stay on your own side.' That's the way it was back then. Real prejudiced."

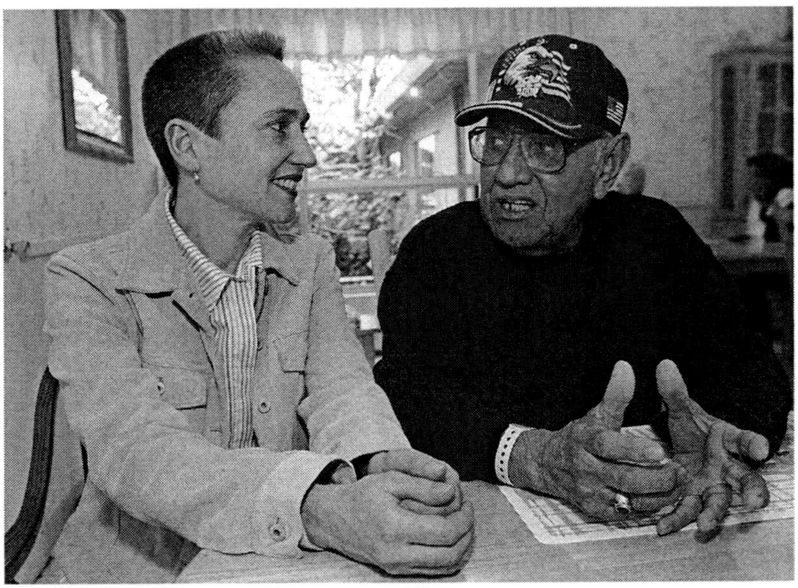

Joe with his writer, Rebekah

Joe takes the conversation another turn, to show that others had it even worse than he did:

"The thing that really got me mad was when I used to live on a ranch and I had to walk to get the bus. I got on and black people tried to get in and the driver said they had to get in the back. I swear to God, I couldn't believe it! They let me in, but the black people had to get in the back! And then this lady, a black lady who was getting on the bus said, 'One of these days we'll be in the driver's seat.'" Joe adds with a tone of defiance, "And she was right."

What matters most, according to Joe's own philosophy, is where he is now and that it is a place of acceptance.

"That must've been painful for you," I say to Joe, "to live with that type of discrimination." Shifting back to the future and his optimistic nature, he answers, "Oh yeah, but there's no discrimination here [at the healthcare center]. They treat everybody the same. That's why I like it here. And if you treat anyone different they'd say something. We're all together. We're here together to stay together and be friends."

Particularly when Joe discusses difficult times from his past that old question of "Who is Joe?" haunts me. At first I wondered if he tried to gloss things over because of my white skin. Maybe he didn't want me to witness his pain or to leave himself vulnerable to me. Perhaps the realization that his story would be published held him back or made him more guarded. Still, the more I meet with Joe, the more I sense a genuineness about him, a quality that reminds me of the people I'm closest to in my own life.

I often wonder how he is able to remain so positive through the racism he experienced as he grew up and in the war. He's shared with me some of his frustration and his anger, but he's always quick to point out that he's "let it go." I hear his voice in my head insisting, "Everything is beautiful now. Right here, it's beautiful."

What would have happened if Joe had actually been given the chance to swim and dive and prove himself? I feel overwhelmed with sadness thinking about those denied opportunities and about Joe's painful past. But then I remember—this is Joe's life and Joe's world and it's he who's chosen to focus on what is most important to him—family, friends and work.

Joe isn't weighed down by his frustration and anger. I don't know, and probably never will, if this is simply who Joe has always been, or if it's a way of being he's mastered over his lifetime. What matters most, according to Joe's own philosophy, is where he is now and that it is a place of acceptance.

One of the hardest parts of life to accept must be his inability to work like he used to. Work, like family and friends, is at the core of Joe's existence. At the nursing home, he still manages to have all three. After a life of working hard, Joe's thankful that work is now allowed rather than required.

Joe worked as a farm worker, migrating between Northern and Southern California each year. In Brawley, his job was sorting and loading watermelons and cantaloupe onto trucks, and sometimes helping in the packing shed. But the work there was more demanding and didn't pay as well as "up North." In Southern California, Joe's salary averaged forty cents an hour, but in the San Jose and the Mountain View area he could easily make more.

One year, when he was finally old enough to live on his own, he decided to stay "up North" rather than returning to Brawley at the end of the season. Besides, he always had friends wherever he was because everyone took the same migration route each year. The children grew up together, eventually married and started their own families.

It was after his move that he met his wife, Gloria, at a dance in San Jose. The best dances, he recalls, were on Sundays at the Civic Auditorium in San Jose, where an orchestra would play throughout the evening. Men were required to dress in suits and ties and women to wear long gowns, unlike the more casual Saturday night dances at the Rainbow.

"It was mostly Mexicans that would go," Joe explains. "Gloria would go and she was always with her cousins. She was a real beautiful dancer. So I went and picked her out and she fit right in my arms," he laughs. "I used to dance pretty good back then. Not so much anymore, but back then I could dance... My brother, Frank, was a dancer so I'd go peek on him and watch him dance. He had some wild moves, though. I liked to dance different. I like to swing a girl around when I'm dancing."

After that first meeting at the dance, Joe and Gloria started dating. They lived in different San Jose neighborhoods. "I used to go visit her in the barrio where she lived—Sal Si Puedes. That means 'Get out if you can.'" Joe shakes his head laughing, as he describes what he calls a "real tough neighborhood." Since he was known there, he was able to come and go without any trouble. It was during this time, at the very beginning of the farm workers' movement, that Joe first met the famous activist Cesar Chavez. Though Joe himself was not a part of the movement, he affirms, "I stood behind Cesar. It's hard working in the fields, especially at that time. So what he did was important."

Cesar's brother, Lenny, and Joe were good friends. Joe and Gloria later became *compadres*, or godparents, to Lenny's daughter.

After Joe was married he began working on the Shibuya family's carnation farm in Mountain View, where he would cut and load carnations onto a truck for sale in San Francisco. Eventually, his wife joined him working on the farm, and they moved into a house provided by the Shibuyas until the property was eventually sold. An apartment building and shopping center soon replaced the forty acres of farmland, and the young couple then worked for another Japanese family that had been recommended by the Shibuyas.

Joe's daughter, Teresa, was born in San Jose after work on the carnation farms came to an end. But eventually the marriage ended in divorce. "I don't remember how long I was married," Joe admits, "but it was quite a while. We were real close but it was just one of those things that happen." Teresa stayed with her mother. "She was small when we separated so she didn't know what was up." Joe would visit her and give her money. He's grateful that his wife never said anything bad about him. "For my daughter's sake," Joe tells me.

Still, he has fond memories of Teresa's childhood. "My daughter is real special to me. We were a real close family and we had some good times back then." He recounts a family trip to Disneyland. "She was small and we gave her a doll. She looked just like that doll. And we went on all the rides and she wasn't scared of any of them." He even put her in the water of their hotel pool at Disneyland. "Her grandma was looking down from the balcony shaking her fist at me and grrr," Joe pretends to growl, laughing. "She was looking down at me, like 'What are you doing with that baby?' But Teresa wasn't scared. She was never scared." He leans forward in his chair with a smile across his face as he remembers the name of her favorite doll, Lulu, and says again how fearless his daughter was.

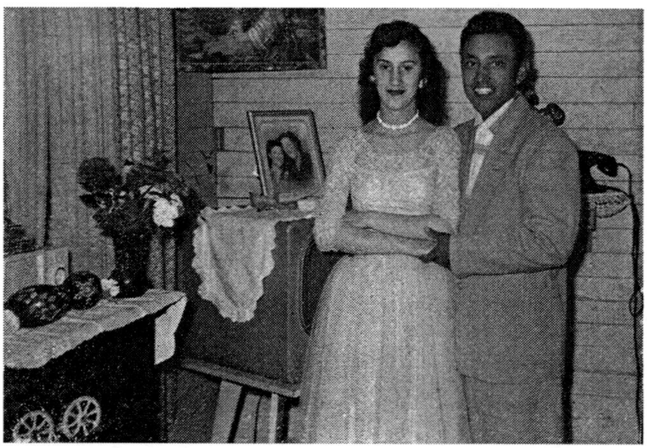

Joe and Gloria in the living room

Like Joe, Teresa likes sports. Their enjoyment of football and baseball games together became another strong bond between them. "My ex-wife let me take her any time. Teresa likes sports, just like me. We're both 49ers fans."

Many of Joe's family memories center around outings. On Easter, the family would spend the day at Alum Rock Park, arriving early to find a prime spot to spend the afternoon swimming and picnicking. We always had a real good time together," Joe tells me.

Fairs in San Jose were also a part of the "good time." The fairs lasted for two weeks and the entire family—Joe, Gloria, Teresa, cousins, brothers and sisters—would go and spend the day together relaxing and having fun. They were special when Teresa was a baby and later when she was grown with a family of her own.

When he speaks about Teresa, his memories often blend. One memory will be of her childhood and the next of her married life. It's almost as though no time has passed at all between her childhood and the present. Over time I realize that there really doesn't seem to be a need to separate the memories. His love for Teresa has remained constant and unwavering throughout the years, and he still feels the same tenderness toward her today as he did when she was a small child.

His love for Teresa has remained constant and unwavering throughout the years, and he still feels the same tenderness toward her today as he did when she was a small child.

One afternoon I join Joe for music appreciation hour at the home. We walk down the hallway together into the activities room where eight or ten other residents sit at tables sipping drinks and enjoying cheese and crackers.

We take our places at a table and quietly listen to classical music playing from a CD player in the corner. Joe hums softly, his head tipping from side to side as if lost in thought. He tells me the music reminds him of the choir at the Cathedral of Faith in San Jose where he used to attend Mass with his family.

"I liked it because it was different kinds of people who went there. And we were together and you could feel the friendship." Joe pauses, listening to the music for a few seconds before he continues. "The choir sang real beautiful and then you'd hold hands with your neighbor and that's really something. There were all colors, you know— Mexicans, Americans, Chinese and everything. And when you can hold hands with all kinds of people, you can't beat that. At that time you couldn't do things like that. Remember the different races weren't that close, but there we were. It's beautiful. I get chills thinking about it. I do," Joe laughs nodding his head once again to the music.

Joe regularly attended Mass every Sunday with his wife and daughter and he continues the tradition at the nursing home. Each Sunday a priest visits the residents in their rooms and gives communion and says Mass for those who are able to attend. Joe appreciates that services are also available for people of other religions.

"It doesn't matter that it's not my regular church," he tells me. To me, it's still church and I can pray my own way. Everyone can."

After Joe and his wife separated, he moved into an apartment with his sister, Anita, in Mountain View, where he lived until coming to his current home at Mountain View Healthcare Center. He never remarried.

"My ex-wife, she got married after a long time," Joe tells me. "My daughter asked if I was mad and I said, 'No, why should I be?' We made peace and everything. So they got married and I went to the wedding. He was a real nice guy. We shook hands and everything. You got to let people go their own way. But I never wanted to get married again."

Eventually Joe left the fields and worked with his friend, Johnny Martinez, at PG&E for eighteen years doing a variety of jobs. He cleared brush to make way for the electrical towers and later prepared for their installation. Joe still remembers all the steps involved in the dangerous work. The men would dig four holes for each tower and then send another man down to clear them out. It was Joe's duty to clear out the holes, since he was short and could easily move around. Before he went down to work, he was fitted with a protective shield in case the hole collapsed. Later another crew would come to build the towers.

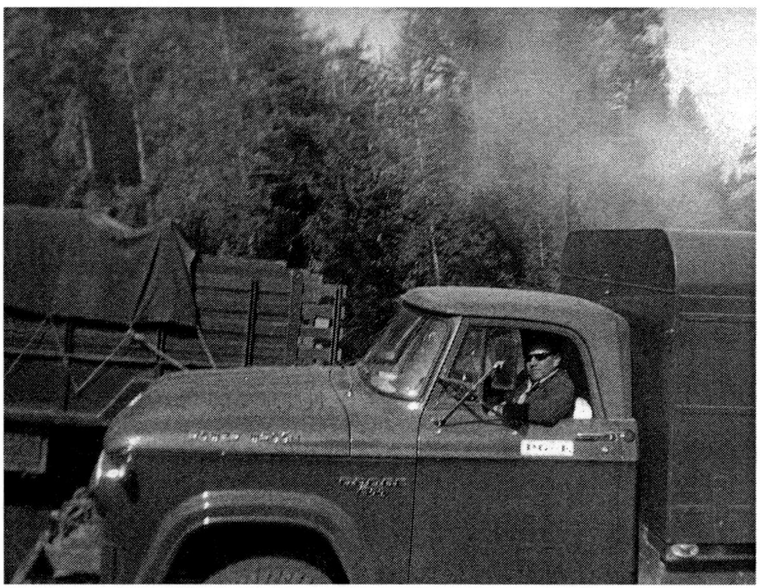

Joe in his PG&E truck

"My *compadre*, Johnny Martinez, did that job because he could climb. He wasn't scared. He asked me to do it and I said 'no way.' But he couldn't do what I did because he was scared to go down. I told him he could keep his job," Joe laughs. "And he told me he wouldn't take my job for nothing. It was okay, though, because even if the hole collapsed you were safe because of the shield. Everyone was scared to go in there except for me."

Joe also worked at a seed processing plant in Morgan Hill and at Syntex, where he cleaned test tubes and later became a janitor when the company began laying off workers. Joe relays the details of all his jobs with the same level of passion and enthusiasm. It's obvious that regardless of the job, Joe has always taken pride in his work.

"I get three meals a day here, I work, and I take good care of myself."

During all of his working years, Joe also volunteered his time doing community service. His former coworkers at Mountain View Community Services still send him notes and cards filled with good wishes, asking if he plans to return. His giving spirit is still evident when he tells me he wants to go shopping when his daughter visits so he can buy beach balls to use during exercise class.

"I want to get some candy, too because I have a big jar that used to be filled up, but it's empty now. The workers here, they love chocolate. And they do everything for us, so I tell them 'If you want some candy, it's right there.'"

Joe attributes his current good health to living at the home. He tells me that when his old friends visit him they hardly recognize him. "'You don't look seventy-seven.' That's what everyone says. But that's what you get for working and staying healthy and eating right." He adds matter-of-factly, "I get three meals a day here, I work, and I take good care of myself."

It's hard for many of his old friends, as it initially was for me, to understand why such a cogent, youthful elder would want to live in a nursing home. Joe has a ready answer, which also explains who he is:

"People ask me, how come you're here? Instead of explaining, I say, 'Oh, I just like it.' Always being on the go, go, go. At least now I'm helping. Somebody put me here for that purpose. And they say, 'Are you gonna go or are you gonna stay here?' And I say, 'I'm gonna stay here.' 'Cause I help them. There's one way or another way to help them. And they thank me. They say, 'Thank you for all your help.' He looks at me pensively, "That's all the money I need, right? That's all the money I need." ■

Joe at Home

a poem by Rebekah Eppley

Some people in the nursing home
talk to themselves
or play cards to pass the time.
Some never see the sunlight
sifting through the window slats
but feel warm nonetheless
and smile in their sleep.
Others wander the halls on stiff legs
braced against a walker
while yet others come to convalesce,
a temporary pass until they return
to lives never quite the same.

Joe is the one who comes for recovery
but remains by choice
rearranging his idea of home.
He never knew there were places like this
where family is what you choose
and work is not required but allowed
and paychecks of thank you cover the cost.
Where roadside help is redirecting
a wheelchair-bound man
temporarily trapped between chair and door,
extending his hand toward the glass
separating August's heat from cool forced air.

On Fridays a musician visits
and how she makes that fiddle cry.
Music lifts him to the old cathedral
where all kinds of people held hands—
Christ it was beautiful.
He says those things didn't happen back then,
says remembering now seems like the way
it always was
was meant to be
even though we were taught different truths
and the unknown was what we feared.

He says back then we were separate always
the racial divide sliced through the center
so they kept their ways and we kept ours.
And there were things I wanted
wanted so bad,
but chances all came from that other side.
I knew how to work and made good money
had what I needed and made my way.
But here at home, those memories elusive
we take care of each other
and it's the life that you make.

May 2, 2005

WRITER'S PROFILE

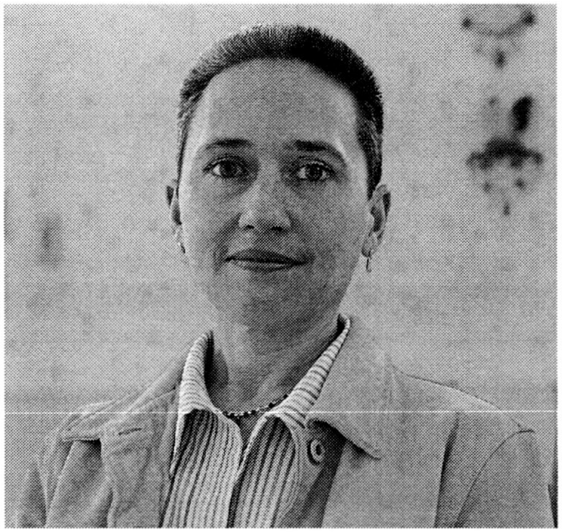

Rebekah Eppley

In college I used to visit a nearby nursing home and write letters for the residents whose fingers could no longer hold a pen or who had lost use of their hands. While the pretext for my visit was to help the seniors accomplish a task, I soon realized that they were eager for conversation and wanted to share their stories. I, in turn, was a willing listener and welcomed the companionship of an older person. My grandfather was in the late stages of Parkinson's and Alzheimer's disease when I was a child. I grew up reading letters and stories he wrote to my mother when she was young. Through those accounts captured on paper, I was able to learn about my grandfather and find a connection with him through his humor and imagination.

For the past ten years I have worked in fundraising for the Institute on Aging while also earning a Master's Degree in Creative Writing. While my work usually happens in an office, a favorite part of my job has been interviewing seniors for newsletter articles or special projects and learning more about their histories.

As a fiction writer I'm always looking for stories, collecting tales to find my way towards some larger truth. I entered this project while also writing a collection of prose poems about Mexico based on stories that had been told to me. I often struggled with how to tell these accounts that had been handed down, how to stay true to their essence. Working with Joe has helped me to step aside so that I can hear them in a new way.

I'm thankful for the opportunity to learn about Joe through his recollections. I would often leave our sessions filled with vivid images of his childhood in the fields or of Joe as a young man, spinning a partner across the dance floor. During the course of our meetings, Joe became a teacher to me, imparting a wisdom I hope to have as I grow older. From our meetings, I'll carry with me Joe's definition of home as a place where there are friends, where there is mutual respect and where "we take care of each other."

HELEN RAND PARISH

Willow Tree Nursing Center
Oakland, California
with
Kathleen Barrows

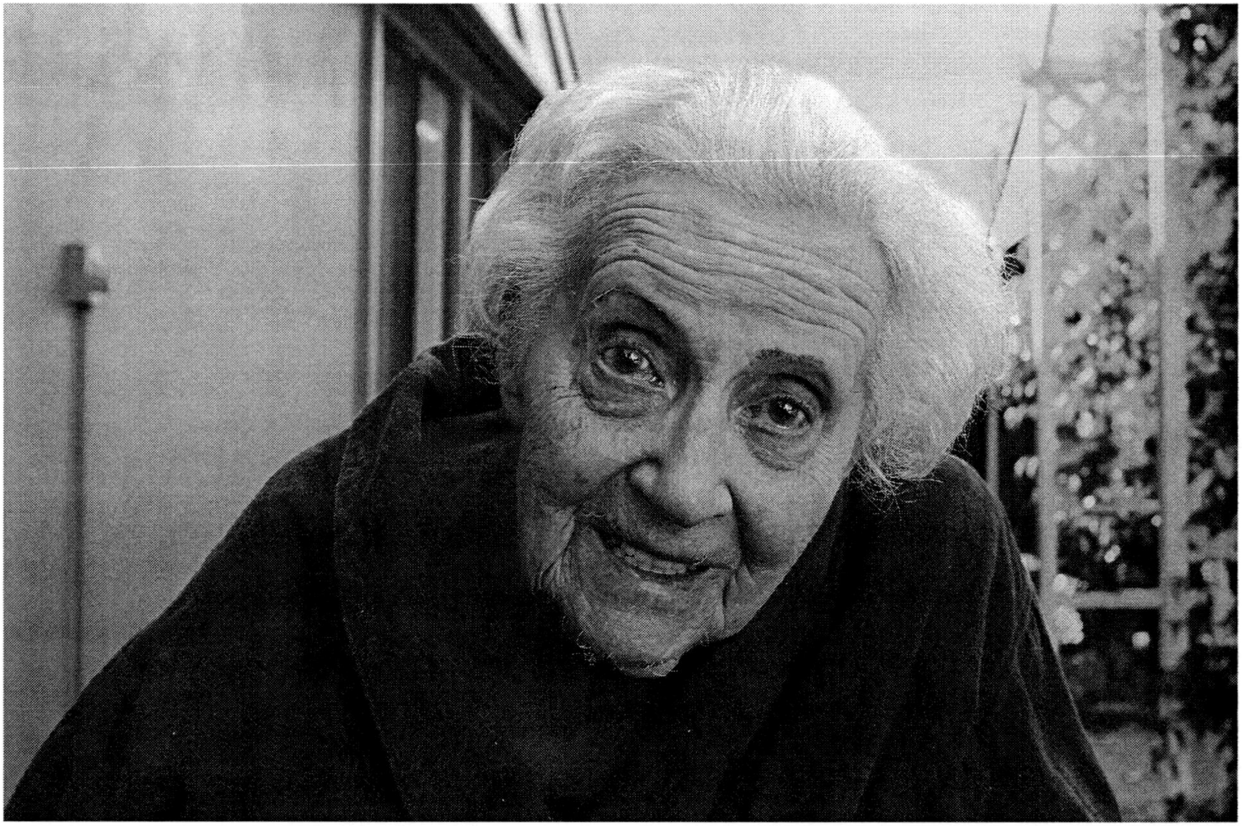

"I was born a tuffy"

"I have a tale to tell, the like of which men have never heard before." So begins Helen Parish's book for young adults, the account of Estebanico, an African slave who was part of the ill-fated Spanish expedition in search of the Seven Cities of Cibola nearly five centuries ago.

I sit here in the silence of Bancroft Library at UC Berkeley, surrounded by gold-framed paintings, graying professors and young college students tapping on their notebook computers or shuffling through cardboard boxes of documents. I've traced Helen's steps, to the dark and dingy alcove on Tier 5 of the renowned library where Helen did much of her work as a research associate. Her spirit, right now, sits like a ghost in the empty chair beside me as I open the pages to her book *Estebanico.*

"That is the way it used to be when kings told their story," she explains. Then I'll be your scribe, I respond.

Today, almost nine months after first meeting Helen, the task of relating a tale, "the like of which men have never heard before," weighs heavy upon me. (Helen, of course, were she relating her own story today, would correct it for modern times to say "Men *and* women.") Many years ago, when she was researching the life of the sixteenth century Spanish priest and social reformer, Bartolomé de las Casas, the nuns in the convent where she was staying asked who would go through her archives. Now decades later, I respond to their question, heavy with a sense of responsibility, "It's me." Helen has confirmed, "Yes, it's you."

She's come up with a possible title for her memoirs: *The Thrilling Life Story of Helen Rand Parish as Told to Kathy Barrows*. "That is the way it used to be when kings told their story," she explains. "Then I'll be your scribe," I respond.

This is the story of Helen Rand Parish as told to Kathy Barrows, and the tale of how Helen Rand Parish and Kathy Barrows came to become good friends. It is the tale of a brilliant and witty writer, scholar and community activist who welcomed a new friend into her life at a very old age and of how they learned together the miracle of coincidence.

August 2004, Ashby Care Center, Berkeley

After just a few visits, I've come to realize that Helen, at ninety-one, serves as the guardian of the door of this long-term care facility. Today she sits in her wheelchair, bundled in an afghan of primary colors, her feet snuggled in flowered slippers, her lips aglow with red lipstick. She's

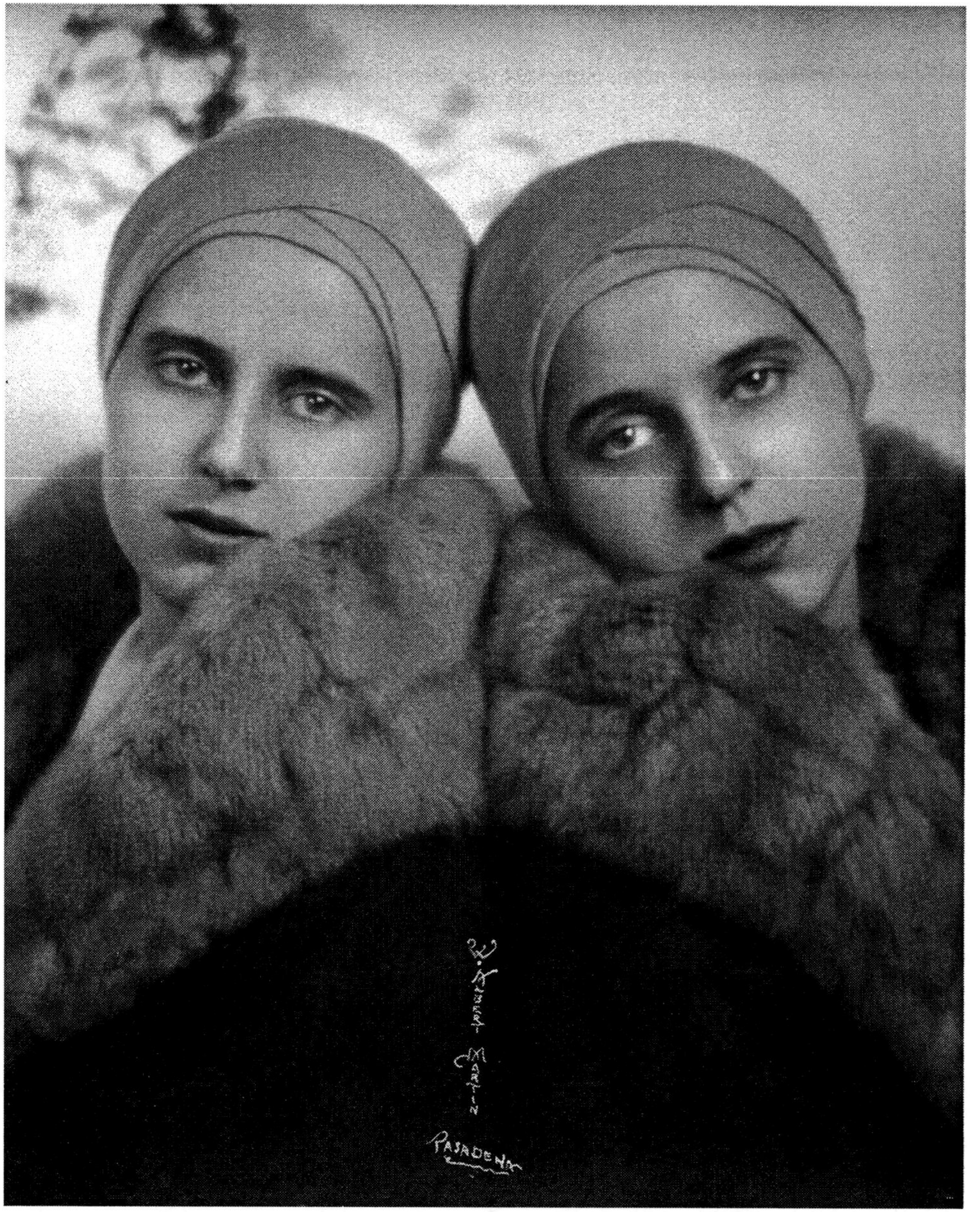

Helen and her identical twin Olive

looking through the large entry window toward an unknown place beyond the concrete parking lot and street clogged with cars. Her eyes are grayish blue, emphasized by arched eyebrows that vary in color from green to copper, depending on the day and the nurse who has painted them on. Her white hair, thinning just a little, has enviable waves; her nose, long and sharp, I like to think of as a "detective nose"—the one she's followed throughout her life to track down the mysteries of other people's lives.

On the rare days when I find her sitting with her fellow residents in the "living room," her diminutive, four-foot-eleven, 110-pound frame is almost invisible. Her shoulders bend forward as she sometimes struggles to catch her breath, which is precious to her these days. Often her conversation is punctuated by audible wheezing. "It's not *pneu*monia (*new*monia)," she quips; "it's *old*monia," referring to the chronic bronchitis and a leaking heart that have plagued her since childhood.

"It's not *pneu*monia (*new*monia)," she quips; "it's *old*monia," referring to the chronic bronchitis and a leaking heart that have plagued her since childhood.

Helen doesn't like to sit in her room; it's a large dark room, the curtain often drawn on the window. Four beds line one wall, with simple but pleasant matching flowered bedspreads. Her space is easily identifiable. Books rest on her bed stand and bureau, and on her altar rest Tibetan cymbals *(Tingsha)* and photos. A portrait of Helen peers out over her bed. She's in her twenties, stylishly dressed with a fur collar. Her head is covered with a turban and she is leaning in toward a mirror image of herself...

October 10, 1912, Waterbury, Connecticut

Helen and her identical twin, Olive—the mirror image in the photo—were born on October 10, 1912, in a double breech birth, in Waterbury, Connecticut, near New Haven. Helen talks about her birth as if she remembers it, and after many visits with her, I've almost come to believe she does. "I was on top so I came out with my fist," she says, holding up a clenched fist. "We came out at the same time...I was born a toughie; that's *t-u-f-f-y* [spelling out the word]. My mother was a tuffy, too. She was the *real* heroine." Helen then launches into her theory about the origins of her mother: that she was a gypsy, born in Belarusia and switched at birth into a French family. Her mother's heritage, she says, can be proven by her gypsy habit of consuming eight glasses of water a day.

When Helen talks of her "tuffy" status, as she does frequently, she inevitably adds, "My nephew, Rick, is a semi-tuffy. *He* takes naps." It's he,

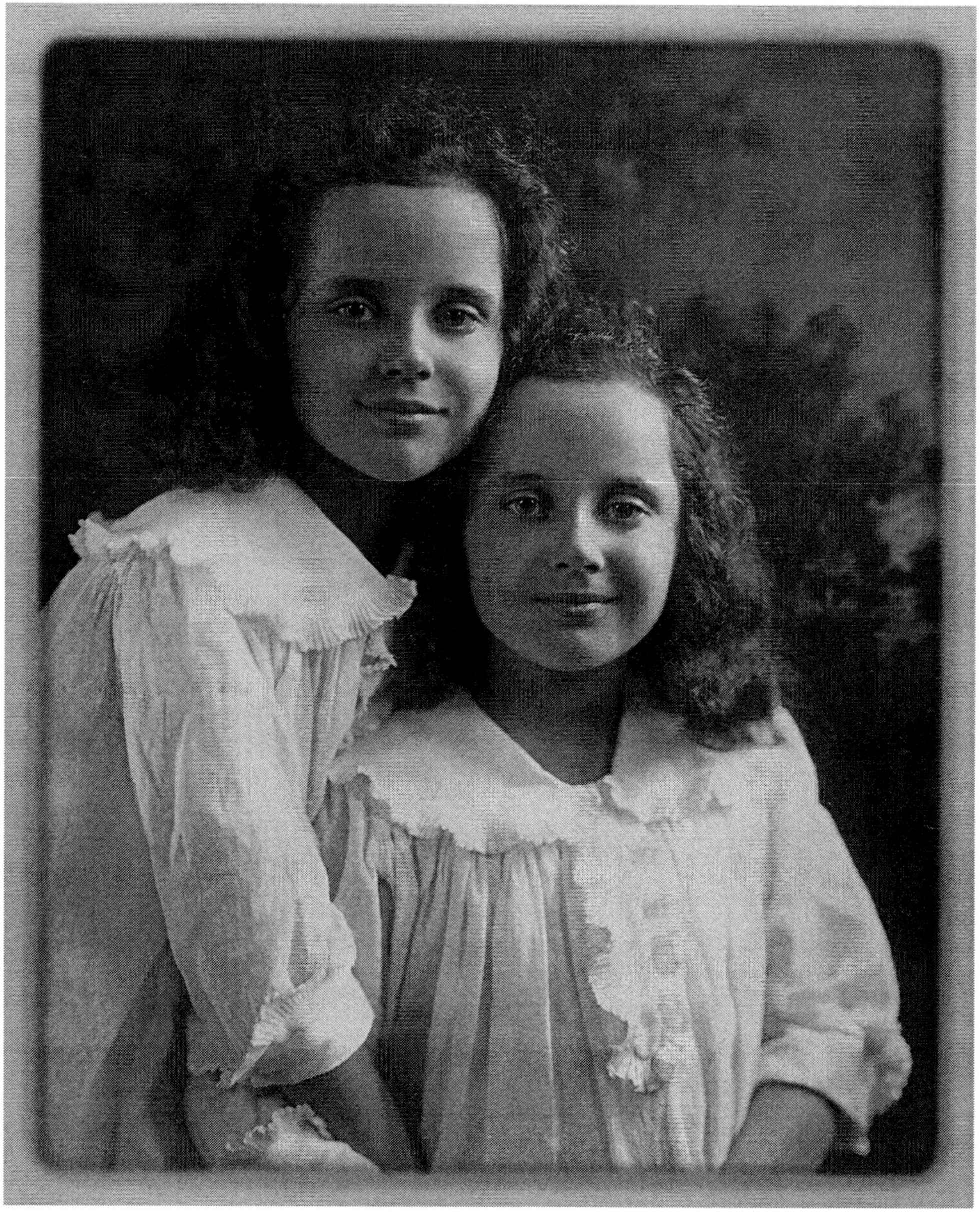

The young Parish twins

the second son of Helen's twin sister, who provides an alternative explanation of his grandmother's origin. After considerable research, Rick posits that Helen's mother, Olive Helene Slade, was born in the Ukraine of a family of Jewish descent that later fled the Jewish pogroms of 1886 and settled for awhile in Paris. The family immigrated to the United States around the turn of the century. Helen's mother considered herself French and brought up the twin girls with French as their first language.

"The rich have their heads on backwards. I never thought like a rich person."

The year of their birth is another small point of contention between Helen and Rick. Following a tradition of Eastern cultures, Helen prefers to view the year of conception as the "real birthday," the beginning. "This is Chinese style. When you're born, you're a year old and the next time when it's January 1, you're two years old," she explains. Finally, she concludes, "So I'm really going to be ninety-three."

The twins were raised by their parents in a grand thirty-room home, complete with a governess, servants and horses for the girls to ride. Helen describes her family as "filthy rich, dangerously rich," adding, "The rich have their heads on backwards. I never thought like a rich person." Her father graduated as a metallurgical engineer in the first class of Yale's famous Sheffield Scientific School, where he met his wife, who was majoring in chemistry. According to Helen, at that time marriage between students was prohibited. "Yale was a very bigoted place. And my father and my mother, they defied the rules. There would be God knows what punishment if they were caught, but they weren't caught. They made a perfect pair," she asserts.

Albums of childhood photos, all scrupulously collected and saved by their mother, chronicle the privileged life of the twins and the changing styles of the times. The twins dressed as flappers, with marcelled hair, at a ball on a transatlantic steamer after a trip to Europe—always mirror images of each other. Few would notice Olive's slight eye defect from a childhood accident or her narrower face. As Olive's son Rick points out, one's always laughing and the other isn't, but to this day he's not always sure which one appeared the merrier.

The twins became research subjects for the famous American psychologist Arnold Gesell, founder and director of the Clinic of Child Development at Yale, and appeared in an early *Scientific American* article authored by the pioneer in child psychology. Helen loves to recount one of the many "tests" he administered to the twins when they were eight: "You'd have to tell your favorite book and my sister put 'stories from the Bible,' and *I* put 'the Bible.' Obviously, it's the same thing, but *I* put it differently," she adds in a tone of sisterly competition. "Pretty damn good, as the British would say!" Later, shortly before their graduation from college at the age of sixteen, the twins were placed in a separate room, given pencils and papers, and told to draw three images. Both twins drew identical items: a tree, a carriage and a baby.

Bilingual in French and English from early childhood, by eight they had added Spanish to their repertoire, on the insistence of their Cuban-born grandmother, Juana Rand Parish. It must have been a challenging task to be teacher of such a precocious pair. In elementary school, the twins simply switched to French when they were scolded for talking too much, and if the teacher was called out of class while reading a story, one of the twins would take over the reading for her.

Though the father is obscure at best, according to Helen he died when she was nine years old, leaving her mother to raise the twins.

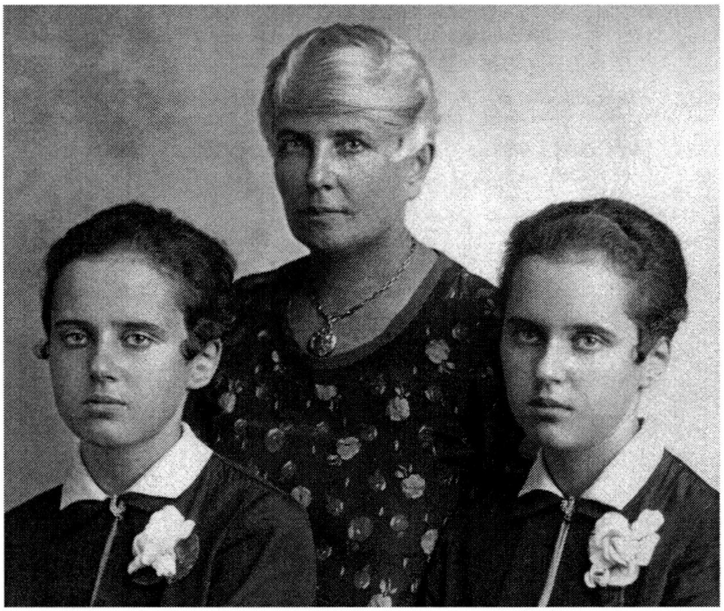

The young Parish twins with their mother

1920s, Atlanta, Georgia

The twins' enrollment in Oglethorpe College took them and their mother to Atlanta. They were fourteen at the time. College President Thornwell Jacobs was shocked, according to a 1928 *Atlanta Constitution* article, when "two small girls, still in socks, big curls and sailor hats," approached him with their mother for early admission to the well-regarded southern college. But he needed no convincing after the twins' near-perfect scores on the entrance exams. At fifteen, they became college correspondents for the *Atlanta Constitution*, their articles, always accompanied by their picture and signed with the by-line "The Parish Twins."

After graduating from Oglethorpe College in 1928 with summa cum laude honors in Greek and Latin, they returned with their mother to Connecticut. There they graduated from Yale a year later, at the age of seventeen, with their master's degrees in American literature and history.

By 1929 they were back in Atlanta, where their witty columns for the front page of the newspaper's second section became the talk of the town. An article that year in the *Atlanta Constitution* described the famous seventeen-year-old "reporterettes": "The twins are endowed with superior intellect, but with all their knowledge are filled with the joy of life and possess a remarkable sense of humor...[Their] personality is blended so perfectly that they seem rather to be one person than two."

"The twins are endowed with superior intellect, but with all their knowledge are filled with the joy of life and possess a remarkable sense of humor..."

Helen and Olive quickly advanced to become theater editors at the Georgian paper, developing friendships with musical celebrities such as Feodor Chaliapin. So impressed was he by the account of his backstage make-up session that the famous Russian opera bass insisted that on a return trip the pair meet him at the train station. On their first assignment for the *New York Daily Mirror*, where their by-line changed to "The Mirror Twins," New York Mayor Jimmy Walker was so enthralled with the idea of twin reporters that he switched roles and interviewed *them*.

But Helen and Olive weren't just twins. Always accompanied by their mother, they were part of an inseparable trio. Olive Helene became a ghostwriter, and the three frequently collaborated on stories, gaining the name "Les Trois Parishes." Thinking Lestrois Parish was a male journalist, confused editors unfamiliar with French would send them boxes of cigars.

The three traveled and lived together for years. In Los Angeles the twins pursued post-graduate work at UCLA, and studied agrarian law in Mexico City, while freelancing for the *New York Times*. Eventually they settled in Berkeley, where the twins studied with the famed Latin American historian Herbert Eugene Bolton.

But soon Les Trois Parishes was

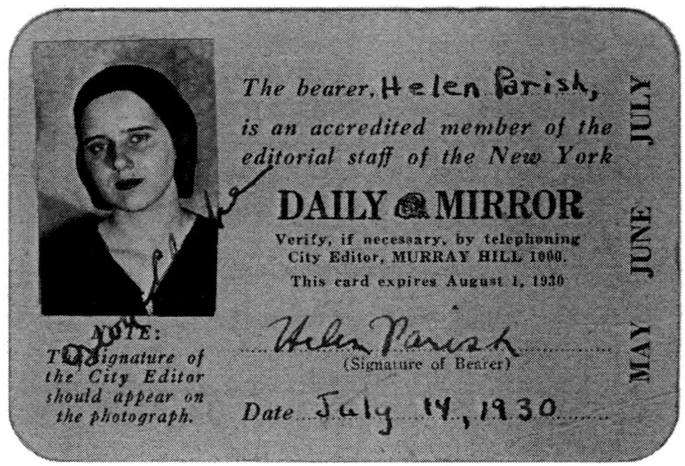
The bearer, Helen Parish,
is an accredited member of the editorial staff of the New York
DAILY MIRROR
Verify, if necessary, by telephoning City Editor, MURRAY HILL 1000.
This card expires August 1, 1930
Helen Parish
(Signature of Bearer)
Date July 14, 1930
NOTE: The Signature of the City Editor should appear on the photograph.
JULY JUNE MAY

Helen's press card, 1930

reduced to a pair when Helen's sister married Hernan Tejada-Flores, the oldest son of the former Bolivian President, Jose Luis Tejada Sorzano. She and her husband later settled in Pasadena, where she had four children and continued on her own path.

Today, Helen talks little of her twin sister, who died in 2001. "Every time I talk about her I cry," she admits, "and I don't want to cry." In more candid moments, when I ask her how it felt to be a twin, she'll confess, "We were freaks." Yet, when I inquire when the happiest time of her life was, she'll respond, "my childhood."

Today, Helen talks little of her twin sister, who died in 2001. "Every time I talk about her I cry," she admits, "and I don't want to cry."

Helen's Birthday, October 10, 2004, Ashby Care Center

I'm sure Helen must be missing Olive's presence, as she sits quietly observing her ninety-second birthday party today. The "living room" of Helen's small nursing home is bustling with music and activity. Helen, dressed in her favorite color, purple, and sporting a matching beret, is surrounded by friends who wait for a chance to offer a small gift, a card or simply words of congratulations.

Helen's not in a talkative mood today, perhaps lost in thoughts of the past that is so present today here with her friends. Her face brightens with a wide smile when the musical performances begin.

An informal a cappella ensemble, which for years performed in Helen's North Berkeley neighborhood, has been invited by Helen's nephew to serenade her for the occasion with early music and madrigals—Helen's favorite music. Known as the Arch Street Irregulars, the group sang regularly at Helen's apartment. One of the sopranos in the group still remembers the first time they met, when Helen, enchanted by their Christmas caroling on the street below, threw open the window of her upstairs apartment and invited the group up for refreshments. The invitation started a tradition of home concerts, the last one in Helen's apartment in 2001.

Many of the friends who come today—and still visit her regularly at the nursing home—have attended those concerts in a very different setting.

1940-1999, Thornburg Village, Berkeley

Helen lived for over half a century in a famous North Berkeley architectural landmark, Normandy Village, just a few steps from campus. The complex features a large stone archway that welcomes guests into a medieval world of cobbled sidewalks, hidden streets, and winding stone staircases that disappear into heavy wooden doors. It's bounded on one side by a jagged picket fence, which has the look of having been constructed some dark night by a band of Irish faeries. One of the pickets, which is topped with the silhouette of a witch, was carved for Helen at the request of a neighbor.

Built in the 1920s by William Yelland, master of the "storybook style" of architecture so frequently associated with Carmel, the village was commissioned by World War I flying ace Col. Jack Thornburg. The original eight-unit block of the "village," where Helen lived, was named after him. The set of buildings was planned as a self-sustained complex where students and faculty could live together in community.

For over a decade I had walked by the whimsical village, tempted to peek in a window where I imagined cave-like rooms lit by candles. The first of our many "co-innocences," Helen's word for "coincidences," came the day we realized we had lived right down the street from each other. I had lived in the top floor of an ugly modern building overlooking San Francisco Bay, while Helen was tucked away in a small apartment in Thornburg Village.

The first of our many "co-innocences," Helen's word for "coincidences," came the day we realized we had lived right down the street from each other.

Helen and her mother lived in the second floor of the building, which was adorned with a fading painted image of a Gallic rooster, one of the national symbols of France—a perfect match for the French-speaking pair. In my search to follow in Helen's footsteps, I climbed the steep curving stairway to Helen's old apartment. Hand-carved by the architect on her dark-stained redwood door is a stanza from the Rubaiyat of Omar Khayyam. It begins:

> "And as the Cock crew, those who stood before
> The Tavern shouted—'Open then the door!"

But I was reluctant to knock on the door and instead visited the Berkeley History Room of the Berkeley City Library to help recreate Helen's life in the village. There, librarians still speak fondly of Helen, recalling her frequent phone calls to the reference department that were always initiated with the same question, "With whom am I speaking?" And as they did with Helen, they lead me to articles that help to answer my questions.

I step, in my mind, through her redwood door and see the image of the apartment's interior as it was when Helen and her mother lived there—

complete with furnishings appropriate to the historian Helen was. An ornate Peruvian sixteenth-century wooden chest, inlaid with scenes of Incan monarchs and bullfighting Spaniards, decorated Helen's small, cluttered study, with triple-latticed windows supplying the only natural light. A nineteenth-century Russian icon hung from the wall and a seventeenth-century carved and gilded altar set the atmosphere of the two-story living room, with its high-peaked ceilings of exposed redwood panels and beams and a tall brick fireplace. Upstairs, in the loft that served as Helen's and her mother's bedroom and as the "stage" for many of the Arch Street Irregulars' biannual concerts, an encapsulated fragment of a 700-year-old manuscript of St. Thomas Aquinas hung on a prayer chair.

"Oh, she was great! I would listen to her for three hours and every word was interesting; maybe I would say ten words, and it would be a delightful afternoon."

A longtime friend brings Helen into the scene:

> "When I think of Helen, I see her in her living room, sitting in her chair by her desk, in this beautiful kind of dark French-style room, with the antiques, the throw rugs, and real wood furniture, and old lamps and everything old and antiquey—another era. She's with her typewriter and books, and stacks of papers all around, surrounded by the paraphernalia of her trade. She's reaching for a book and putting it back and talking and reminiscing... In her day she could spin a yarn. Oh, she was great! I would listen to her for three hours and every word was interesting; maybe I would say ten words, and it would be a delightful afternoon."

The papers, she adds, Helen always held together with straight pins, not paper clips or staples.

Helen and her mother moved to the Berkeley complex in the early '40s, after Olive's marriage. They cared for each other until her mother's death at the age of ninety-two, though Helen will always claim that it was Olive Helene who cared for her. She often told the story of her mother's unusual habit of lifting hard-boiled eggs from boiling water with her bare hands. When Helen asked why she did it, her mother, who did all the cooking, responded, "Because I can." It was she who also seemed to be responsible for Helen's captivating smile. Helen liked to recount a childhood memory when she came down the stairs dressed for school. Her mother commented that she wasn't dressed yet. When Helen asked what was missing, Olive Helene explained, "You're not wearing a smile."

Helen speaks frequently of her mother's talents in the kitchen. I can imagine Olive Helene cooking up one of her French culinary delights for dinner with one of their dearest friends, the Irish poet and folklorist Ella Young. While she did the cooking, Ella and Helen gathered around the table in lively conversation. Maybe they were chatting about one of what Helen says were Ella's four favorite things in life: books, politics, friends and gardening. When she speaks of Ella, Helen often recites a stanza from another Irish poet, Thomas Moore:

"The harp that once through Tara's halls
The soul of music shed
Now hangs as mute on Tara's wall
As if that soul were fled."

Over the years, Helen became the matriarch and oldest resident of Thornburg Village, befriending her neighbors in the complex, all of whom were decades younger than herself. She would invite them to tea in the afternoons and enlist their help to run errands. She and her mother planted a tree in the courtyard, and it was in part through Helen's efforts that the complex was designated a Berkeley historical landmark. It was with the assistance of neighbors and the help of home-care aides that she was able to live there as long as she could. But eventually failing health and finances took her to Ashby Care Center.

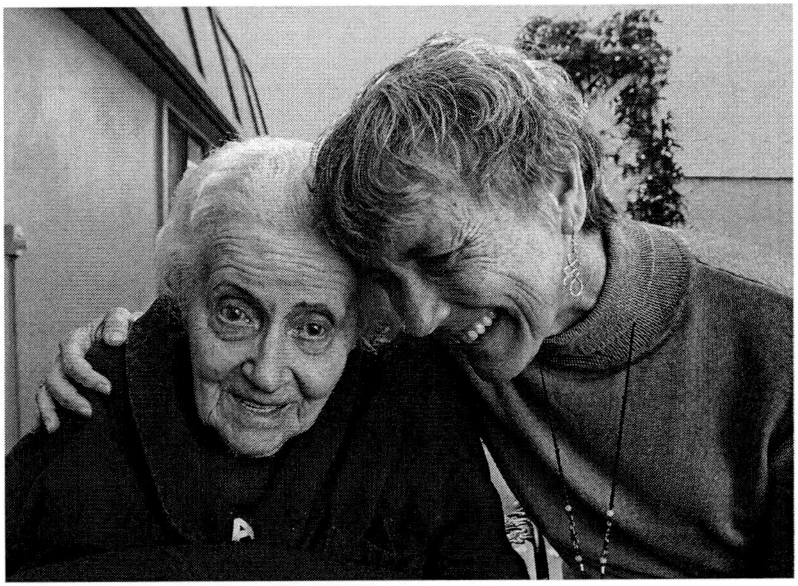

Helen with her writer, Kathleen

Helen admits that the hardest thing in her life has been living in a nursing home. When I ask her, what's the second hardest, she responds gravely, "There is no second hardest." And what gets her through it? "Humor is what allows you to get through all the difficult situations."

Still, Helen is one of the most

frequently visited residents in her nursing home. An old Thornburg Village neighbor drops by at least three times a week, saying Helen is like the mother she never had. Her nephew Rick visits regularly, periodically sneaking her in a treasured cup of coffee, taking her on rare visits to the hairdresser, bringing her library books and hanging new photos on her wall. Helen regales the nurses, physical therapists and residents gathered around the dining room table with her bad jokes and unusual limericks. I often find her using her Spanish to communicate with nurses' aides whom I find in her room, puffing up her pillows or just holding her hand. In her own very unique way, Helen has managed at her present "home" to put together her own "village."

She nods, scrunches up her mouth in a cross between a pout and a smile, crosses her eyes, and looks up at me with affection, replying, "You were sent by heaven."

October 30, 2004, Ashby Care Center

Our mutual fascination with Latin America is our co-innocence of today. Helen and I are sitting together at her spot at the front door and I'm anxious to see her response to a copy of her 1949 children's book, *At the Palace Gates*. It's a book about Paco, the nine-year-old Indian boy from the hill country of Peru, who goes to the capital city of Lima, befriends the llamas at the gates of the presidential palace and eventually saves the President of Peru.

"You told me this was your favorite book, and I was *so* happy to find it," I exclaim as I set the book on her lap. "It's out of print and difficult to find, but good detectives find what they look for. *You* know that. Does this book take you back there?" I ask, as I slowly turn the pages, showing her the illustrations.

"I lived in Lima myself, Helen," I explain, "so I've been to the Plaza de Armas," where much of the action takes place. Helen puts on what I've come to call her "clown face." She nods, scrunches up her mouth in a cross between a pout and a smile, crosses her eyes, and looks up at me with affection, replying, "You were sent by heaven."

1940s, Berkeley

The idea for the children's book, Helen explains in the book flap, originated with her historical interest in colonial street vendors, her visits to Lima, and her correspondence with a nine-year old Peruvian about the beauties of Lima's Plaza de Armas. On the one short vacation she took (Helen prefers to call them "*ve*cations" and today denies that she ever took one), she wrote the final version of the book, which won the Commonwealth Club's Juvenile Book Award in 1948 and was translated into Norwegian in 1962.

The book was illustrated by Leo Politi, the children's book illustrator known for the popular *Madeleine* series. "He was famous and I was an unknown," she admits, but "he was the person that found the right name for the book."

The book was one of three Helen wrote for children or young adults, but she admits that she originally wrote the books with another audience in mind: "You think you know everything. It's a delusion. I wrote what I thought was a good novel, but Viking asked me if I would mind bringing out the book I was doing as a children's book, and I said 'but how would I do it?'" It was Helen's editor and mentor May Massey, a well-known children's book editor for Viking Press, who helped her transform some of her adult research into books for youth. Helen worked for years as a ghostwriter for the famous press.

In her late eighties, she dictated to a long-time friend her ideas for yet another children's book based on her days in counterespionage.

Even now Helen still has books floating in her head. In her late eighties, she dictated to a long-time friend her ideas for yet another children's book based on her days in counterespionage. This latest yet unpublished story is narrated by a 276-year-old tortoise, Tui-Malila, that recounts the story of Charlotte, the queen of Tonga, who used the giant tortoise to rest her feet while making her royal decisions. One of those difficult decisions was allowing U.S. ships to hide in the island's main port after the bombing of Pearl Harbor in World War II. The rough story, typed on Helen's ancient manual typewriter by Helen's friend, sits in a purple folder waiting to be polished and published.

2004, Ashby Care Center, Berkeley

Far from the vast worlds—from Peru to Tonga—that Helen has explored in her writings, Helen and I are chatting on the back "patio," a long ten-foot strip of cement at the back of the building. The only signs of nature are a large pine tree, dripping with pinecones and a few flowering plants. I sit in my usual seat, another wheelchair abandoned in the hall and often the only available seating for visitors.

Inspired by a course I'm auditing on Aging and the Human Spirit, I've resolved to ask Helen about how her concept of religion and spirituality has

Despite her spirituality, religion is not so sacred as to escape her infamous "bad jokes."

changed over the years. It's been a hard few weeks as I've listened to Helen's conversation wander between fond memories frequently repeated and statements that travel from the Spanish Inquisition to the present day in the span of a single sentence. My professors have suggested that sometimes spirituality provides a unifying thread in the tapestry of memories in elders' minds.

Helen's room is filled with a mixture of Tibetan Buddhist and Catholic symbols. A large colorful image of Our Lady Of Guadalupe hangs above an altar where Tibetan cymbals lie, and above her bed is a labyrinth and image of a Buddhist woman, Lama Tsering, who lives in Brazil. It's yet another of our co-innocences. I lived in Brazil for ten years, though unaware of the spiritual leader.

When I first met Helen, I wondered if she had been a Catholic nun, as she mentioned in passing that she had taken the vows of "chastity, poverty and obedience." That theory quickly disintegrated when I find her one day reciting a mantra with an old Buddhist friend, a long-time neighbor at Thornburg Village who visits regularly. The religious articles in her room, it seems, are an embodiment of her ecumenical nature.

Despite her spirituality, religion is not so sacred as to escape her infamous "bad jokes," like this one, that peppered her conversation: "There was a discussion between Jesuits, Dominicans and an ordinary citizen. The three of them got together and they couldn't understand which God loved the most. So they asked God to answer them and He sent back a message on a piece of paper and it said, "I love you all, signed, God, S.J."

Helen is delighted when I understand the punch line. As a graduate of a Catholic Jesuit university, I immediately recognize the S.J. initials, indicating that God was a Jesuit.

I myself am what Catholics call "fallen-away." I listen to more dharma talks than sermons and frequent my meditation bench much more than I do the Catholic church, where I attend a yearly Christmas Mass with my still-very-Catholic mother. But I find myself feeling like a disciple listening to a "Sermon on the Mount" as I sit at the foot of her wheelchair while she responds with impressive coherence and eloquence to my question about her spiritual life: "I remember asking my mother on a nice day like this. I was nine years old. And I had said to her 'Tell me about God. What is that?'" Helen goes on to explain that "the question in this case was not who is God; it was what is God. It's a power and above all it is our relation to that power and it stretches as far as we can stretch it." She extends her hand across her lap to indicate the distance.

She then launches into a parable about Diego Rivera, the famous Mexican muralist: "Diego Rivera heard two men arguing about the deity. He was so shocked, he said, 'Thank God, I'm an atheist' because he thought it was stupid to argue about something that you could only guess about." She interprets, "What he meant was 'I don't narrow the concept of God to some little thing. It's an infinite thing and the bigger you can grasp it, the better.'"

From her wheelchair, Helen points toward the trunk of the large pine tree: "Look at the roots. Those are the tree. And if you've ever seen the squirrels run up it, you come close to understanding what is God. You get it? God is not this person or that person; that's a *cramped* perception. If you have this 'Thank God I'm an atheist,' you're touching the edge of the right way."

As Helen and I discuss her philosophy of God, there's a parallel conversation going on in the background. A representative of a Bible-based church denomination is talking with another younger resident of the nursing home, the one who always asks departing visitors for their prayers or a cigarette. While Helen talks of the relativity of God, their talk centers on the truth of the Bible and the devil's battle for man's soul. I leave thinking how the larger conflicts and questions in the world get played out on a different scale here and wishing there were more Helens and fewer "cramped perceptions."

Only seven years ago, Helen's ecumenical view of the world had been publicly recognized in one of the highlights of her career.

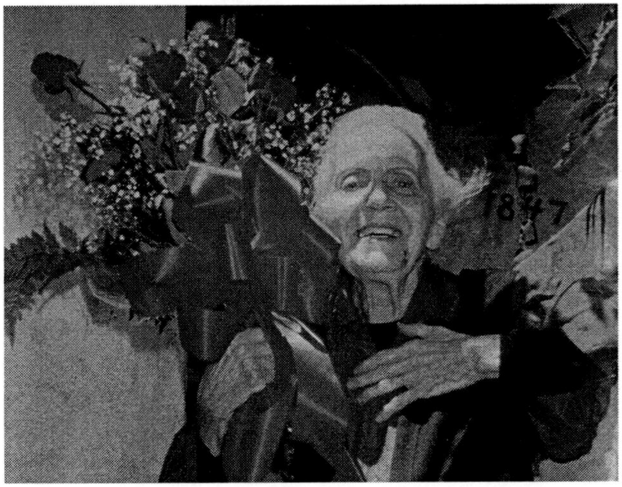

Helen, on the day of her honorary degree, at Thornburg Village

1986, Graduate Theological Union, Berkeley

Helen glowed with excitement as she accepted her honorary doctorate from the Dominican School of Philosophy and Theology. The ceremony took place in the chapel of the Pacific School of Religion on the Graduate Theological Union (GTU) campus. As Helen puts it, "The Dominicans gave me the highest order they can give for a lay person."

"No matter what my research, I get unpublished material that sheds new light. I look in a different place from where everybody else goes."

The degree honored Helen's decades of research into the life and times of Bartolomé de las Casas, a sixteenth-century Dominican priest who spent his lifetime fighting for the rights of the Indians of the New World. In a 1992 interview, she described him as "the only voice in his century to denounce this inhumanity [of the slave trade]." She spent years of her life trying to determine his correct birth date, lobbying for his canonization as a saint, and bringing to Bancroft Library a large collection of rare Las Casas documents. At the age of seventy-nine she was lecturing on Las Casas in Mexico, Spain, and the United States.

Helen frequently refers to him as "my Bartolomé." One day when I mention that at times it sounds like she knew him, she responds, "Well, I know him better than any living person." She never really explains how she got interested in his life, but I learn later that she was inspired by the book of a noted Latin American historian, Lewis Hanke—*The Spanish Struggle for Justice in the New World*. "I didn't choose my work. It chose me," Helen insists.

Las Casas saw his first Indian from the New World as a boy of eight in 1493, in a Palm Sunday procession with Admiral Christopher Columbus. Later, after witnessing firsthand as a planter the exploitation of the Indians, he became their defender. Helen became a world authority on Las Casas' life, authoring numerous books on the subject. Her writing, almost like the style of a historical novel, makes the times come alive, as evident from this excerpt from her classic *Bartolomé de las Casas, The Only Way*, when she was in her seventies:

> "...the town was agog over the return of a crazy Genoese mariner who had just found new lands beyond the ocean sea... Here they came, the prized sight of all: Christopher Columbus in black, his face wind tanned, his eyes hooded; and with him a group of tall, naked, bronze, lean Taino Indians; and his sailors (deloused for the occasion) carrying brilliant red and green parrots, and Indian masks intricately made with tiny shells and beautiful artifacts of beaten gold plates."

That statement, of course, was footnoted to indicate which manuscript in what archive she had gathered the information.

Helen was the meticulous researcher I have always strived to be. With degrees in Spanish and Latin American Studies—in yet another "co-innocence" of our relationship—I had read about Bartolomé de las Casas and spent many a night not in dark archives poring over manuscripts, but at a study desk in the university library. Helen periodically shares her professional secrets with me: "No matter what my research, I get unpublished material that sheds new light. I look in a different place from where everybody else goes." And then adds, "It's great detective work."

It was her research into his life that brought Helen what she terms "the most exciting time of her life." Helen frequently traveled for three months of the year to archives in Spain and the Vatican. Often she'd stay in convents and monasteries. She reminisces about Rome: "My friend Sister Leontina forbade me to go to the early Mass with the sisters. Instead she said I could go up on the roof and watch Rome wake up." I picture her alone on the rooftop of some convent at 4 a.m., her customary time for rising in those days. While nuns in a chapel below chant matins, she waits for the first rays of the sun to glint on a skyline of church domes.

Now, she wakes up every morning with an image of Las Casas greeting her from the wall of her room. The original of the same picture hangs in one of the many Spanish archives where Helen labored unearthing manuscripts on the historical figure.

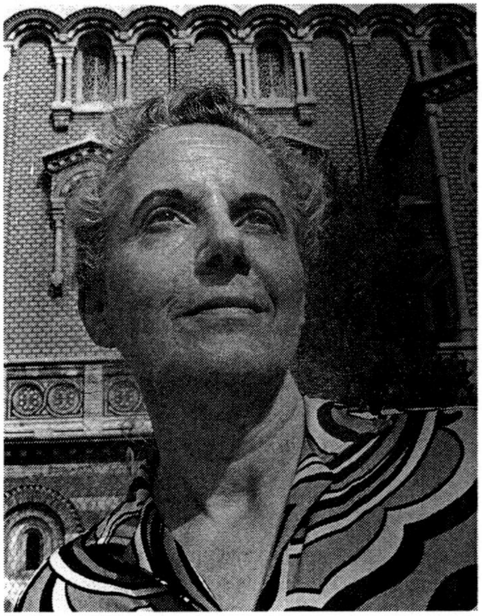

Helen in Italy

November 16, 2005, Willow Tree Nursing Center, Oakland

It's my first visit to Helen's new "home," the day after she has been moved from her old nursing home. It's taken me years—many spent traveling between Latin America and the United States—to finally feel at "home," comfortable in my surroundings. At fifty-six, I find myself reluctant to even think of moving. So what must it feel like to move at ninety-two?

Willow Tree is almost three times the size of Ashby Care Center, though the exteriors look remarkably similar—nondescript one-story facilities, with a drab sixties architectural look and a small parking lot in front. I'm heartened by the banner that hangs above the door: "Ten Years of Caring: 1994-2004" and by the notable absence of employees and residents hanging outside the front door in a haze of cigarette smoke, something I will not miss from Helen's former residence.

Wheelchairs jam the long, wide hospital-like corridors, which are lined with photos of residents in rehabilitation. A loudspeaker summons someone to the nursing station for a telephone call over the beeping of a monitor and the bustle. A helpful nurse directs me to Helen, huddled in her wheelchair, her back to the door. I had walked right past her.

"You're the first person to see me walk," Helen beams, unable to see the tears in my eyes as I trail behind her with a wheelchair should she need to rest.

Helen looks a bit dazed, but she smiles when she sees me. As the nurse shows me the way to Helen's new room, she explains that it often takes elders at least two to three weeks to get used to their new environment. Helen will share her new "home" with her centenarian roommate, Miss Susie, who's sitting in a wheelchair. Both of her legs, covered with a lap quilt, have been amputated above the knee.

Helen's half of the room looks barren right now. Her nephew has lined up on the windowsill her precious belongings—the portrait of Bartolomé de las Casas, an image of Our Lady of Guadalupe, some red and white malla prayer beads and a stunning portrait of Helen herself, with white hair, an angelic smile on her face. Helen tells me a friend painted it. Within a week, it will hang in the hallway outside her door, to identify Helen's space.

A small carton of clothes sits inside her shared closet; a cardboard box of books rests at the foot of her bed. Before I leave, as an exhausted Helen sleeps, I page through one of the books: *Women of Spirit: Stories of Courage from the Women Who Lived Them.* It's signed by a friend, with the inscription: "Live with great spirit." In the weeks to come, I would witness more of Helen's "great spirit."

January 10, 2005, Willow Tree Nursing Center

I find Helen today in Room 7, the physical therapy room, the equivalent of a gym for the old and infirm. She's sitting in her wheelchair with an elastic yellow band around her knees. Pinkie, the physical therapist, sits like a coach on a stool in front of her, counting how many times Helen can inch her stiff knees outward to stretch the band: "18-19, come on Miss Parish, one more." I offer to come back later, but Pinkie insists that I stay and watch. She then rolls Helen's wheelchair close to the parallel bars, where residents, some recovering from surgery, others just trying to keep their bones moving, steady themselves in their slow walk down the "runway" with parallel bars. Pinkie encourages Helen to use her pencil-thin arms to slowly lift herself from her wheelchair, and I sit holding my breath as Helen struggles to steady herself. She grabs on to the rails firmly. Then suddenly she's off, moving her tennis-shoed feet to take twenty small steps.

Like a mother watching her child take her first steps, I watch in amazement. "You're the first person to see me walk," Helen beams, unable to see the tears in my eyes as I trail behind her with a wheelchair should she need to rest. It's the first time I've seen her out of her wheelchair "on her own" in the seven months I've known her, and friends later tell me they're the first steps she's taken in over four years. One, a Thornburg Village neighbor and trekker, thirty years younger than Helen, used to be Helen's walking companion in Berkeley. In those days, the friend says, Helen out-walked her in their urban treks.

"I saw what it was like to raise children and it was a perpetual, unconditional love and I couldn't do it..."

I felt like a mother then, as I do now when Helen needs help drinking her liquid supplements. Ironic that I should feel like a mother to a ninety-two-year-old friend. Yet another co-innocence of our relationship is that neither of us are mothers. When she talks of her sister's marriage and four children, she admits, "I saw what it was like to raise children and it was a perpetual, unconditional love and I couldn't do it... You have to keep on being a good parent all your life. So I saw marriage as a life-long occupation that I didn't want."

Her words echo in my heart. I've never really regretted my decision not to have children—I often heard myself saying the same words. Yet now, at fifty-six, as I care for my eighty-eight-year-old mother, I can't help but wonder who will take care of me.

Helen herself is taken care of by her devoted nephew Rick Tejada-Flores, the second oldest son of Helen's sister who, as Helen once said, "had children for me." Over the months, I've come to realize that it is he and an old friend from Thornburg Village who keep her surrounded with memories of her life. A new photo hanging from the wall or a new library book on her bed stand will always announce one of his frequent visits, as does Helen, who admits how much his visits cheer her up. She just worries sometimes that "he goes too fast."

"Fast"—yes, I've heard that word from my own mother too. "You need to slow down," she'll advise when I complain of a headache. Her requests for my help or company are always preceded with her concern about my hurried schedule. "Do you have time to have lunch with me today?" she'll ask after I've spent a morning running errands with her. Helen's words send messages that even she herself doesn't recognize. But then, Helen has always been a specialist in sending "messages"—most of them very deliberate.

January, 2005, Willow Tree Nursing Center

Ever since the first day we met, Helen has proudly called herself a "passionate pacifist."

"It's nice to go to hell and back if you can help others," rails Helen this afternoon, when we begin our visit. "I don't have to go into politics and fight. We already know there's a crisis. The medical system is a disgrace to this country!" Sifting through the tangled threads of her conversation, seeing her bandaged and black-and-blue wrists from repeated attempts to draw blood, I begin to realize that she has, in the past few days, been taken to the emergency room of a local hospital.

"So you're talking about the care you received when you went into the emergency room?" I ask, trying to clarify.

"I didn't get *any* care in the emergency room," she retorts. "I was there for twenty-four hours and I didn't see a doctor. It's worse than you can imagine... The doctors should go to *jail*. We need to import more South American healthcare workers. How do you like my solution?"

This is not my first glimpse of Helen, the activist. Ever since the first day we met, Helen has proudly called herself a "passionate pacifist." She frequently sports a purple T-shirt, advertising a campaign again domestic violence. And on her wall hangs a poster with the words: "Learn from the world community, cherish the natural order, nurture people, nonconform freely and do justice." The morning after President Bush's inauguration, she exclaims, "Yesterday was the worst day ever for the United States! It's going to get worse everywhere!"

Activism, too, runs in Helen's family. According to Helen's nephew, who co-produced the United Farm Workers' Union (UFW) first documentary film, *Sí Se Puede!*, Helen's mother actually changed her original name to Olive Helene because of her passion for a popular nineteenth-century feminist writer, Olive Schreiner.

But I had never seen Helen this angry. Friends and newspaper articles have filled me in on the details of one example of Helen's activism—at the age of seventy-four.

March 1986, Berkeley City Hall

Armed with neon-colored signs glaring "Dam Texaco Not Strawberry,"

"Save the Swale," and "EIR Now" and a massive store of data, a small grassroots movement of vocal protestors headed by Helen stormed into the Berkeley City Council meeting. Their fight was to prevent the construction of a twenty-eight-unit condominium project at the corner of Hearst and Oxford Streets near downtown Berkeley. The diminutive seventy-four-year old Helen, "clad in violet and black, her grew hair loosely curled in a bun," had to stretch up to the microphone to address the city council, according to a *Berkeley Voice* article on the encounter. Her accusation: "Texaco does not want an EIR (Environmental Impact Report) because they have a dirty and dangerous site."

Helen set up and headed the Oriental section of the Special Security Division (SSD), the counterespionage arm of the Federal Office of Censorship, with headquarters in San Francisco.

Helen, using her detective nose once again, this time for her community, had discovered some files at the Berkeley Police Department. The documentation proved that thousands of gallons of gasoline had leaked into the ground from the pumps of a Texaco gasoline station that had sat for thirty years on the site, located just a block away from Helen's apartment. She also masterminded the slogan, "Save the Swale," though some of the protestors, just like myself, were unfamiliar with the technical term designating a depression in the earth. Helen and her neighbors feared that if the complex were built, the gasoline leakage and the movement of water from a branch of Strawberry Creek could lead to environmental problems, including flooding and soil destabilization.

Helen and her neighbors won the battle against Texaco. To this day, there is an empty lot on the corner of the intersection.

January 15, 2005, Willow Tree Nursing Center

As I turn to enter her quiet, darkened room, so different from the clamor of a Berkeley City Council meeting, I expect to find her sleeping. But instead, I encounter her small figure, looking from the back like some medieval monk bent over a desk while illuminating an ancient manuscript. Light from an old-fashioned desk lamp shines on the book in her hands. Engrossed in her reading, she doesn't stir and as I move around to the front of her wheelchair, she asks that I let her finish the last few paragraphs of the chapter of the book, *Women Who Spied: True Stories of Feminine Espionage,* by A.A. Hoehling. It too holds secrets about Helen's life.

A self-identified "born detective," Helen still uses her detective skills, though on a much smaller scale.

World War II, Berkeley

Though Helen today shrouds her life in counterespionage in secrecy, both from her family and her friends, she did share a few interesting details about her wartime activities with a reporter for the *Oakland Tribune* back in 1968. Helen set up and headed the Oriental section of the Special Security Division (SSD), the counterespionage arm of the Federal Office of Censorship, with headquarters in San Francisco. Working with Latin American governments to intercept espionage communications through postal channels, she was responsible for breaking several important cases.

One was the case of Velvalee Malvena Blucher, documented in the *Women Who Spied* book that I often found sitting on Helen's bed stand. Branded as a "Jap-lover" for her professional and personal involvement with the Nisei community in California, Blucher had fled California with her husband to live in New York in 1937. It seemed that she had used her business as an authority on rare dolls to pass messages to the Japanese government about warship movement on the West Coast. It was Helen who helped decipher the doll-warship code that the spy had created and used in a series of letters to an address in Argentina. Among her discoveries: "New dolls" were actually new warships operating in the Pacific; and a "fisherman with a net" alluded to an aircraft carrier with anti-torpedo nets.

With Helen's detective and linguistic skills (she speaks French, Spanish and Italian, and reads German, Portuguese and some Japanese), she was a natural recruit for the dangerous work. "We were told you don't take the job if you are afraid to be arrested," she recalls. It was hard for me to imagine this passionate pacifist as a spy, but Helen explains, "I felt this was a necessary war and it was good that I could do something... I thought it was wrong for faculty members to go off to war; this was the Second World War, and here I was safe because they had to leave their jobs. So I *had* to do something." But she almost spits out the words when she talks of the "dreadful" J. Edgar Hoover. "He cared more about himself than about anything. He had a rule that you couldn't shake hands with him without wiping your hand with a handkerchief because he didn't like a moist hand."

A self-identified "born detective," Helen still uses her detective skills, though on a much smaller scale. One day we sit in her room studying the robes of her beloved Bartolomé, conjecturing about what season of the year the portrait had been painted. Another day she triumphantly tells me how she figured out the reason for the disappearance of one of the nurses—she was on vacation.

March 2005, Berkeley

I sit at my desk, looking out the window at a neighborhood squirrel swinging like a trapeze artist from the bough of a redwood tree. As I hear him scurry onto my roof with the scratch of his tiny feet, I'm listening to Helen's voice as she relates her concept of God to a squirrel running up a tree.

I've been living and breathing these tapes for weeks, hearing the whir of the tape as it spins through the transcribing machine, modulating the pressure of my foot on the pedal to advance and rewind. The pages of transcription stand as a testimony to our conversations. When I reread them I'm amazed at the mass of words, the advance and rewind of Helen's mind that lies before me—from the Inquisition to modern-day politics, from her simple room in a nursing home in Oakland to the dark archives of convents in Rome. Through the process, I've become the detective that Helen always was, sitting in libraries culling through magazines and newspapers, talking to friends who have known Helen as friend, spiritual mentor and scholar. Some have wept; others laugh and smile. All consider it a privilege to have known her, with many saying she's the most brilliant person they have ever known.

The length of my conversations with Helen, as measured by words spoken, has diminished in the nine months that I've known her. There are long pauses, and I wait patiently for the next word as the tape rolls on. As I listen to her labored breathing, I realize that I can tell when she is smiling, even as she breathes.

As I listen to her labored breathing, I realize that I can tell when she is smiling, even as she breathes.

In our time together, Helen has gone from a self-described "chain-talker" to a quieter person and she now openly admits to her many visitors that she's been demoted to "semi-tuffy" status. Sometimes she forgets to blow me a "sanitary kiss"—when she lifts her fingers to her lips, kisses them and then touches my arm before I leave. I still hope we'll have the time together for her to teach me the latest skill she prides herself on— cheating at bingo.

What is important is that she had the pleasure of remembering and telling her tales, and I had the pleasure of listening to them.

April 28, 2005, Alta Bates Summit Medical Center, Oakland

As I walk through the doors of this Oakland hospital to visit Helen, I suddenly realize that I walked through these same doors thirty years ago, to visit my dying father. I sense that my presence here with Helen today will be the final "co-innocence" of our relationship, and that I've missed my opportunity to play bingo with her.

Helen has been here for four days now, battling a new version of "*old*-monia" and a steadily weakening heart. Her nephew, Rick, reports that on his last visit before she slipped into unconsciousness, she was reviewing family history with him. She has been regaled by the recounting of stories of life in Thornburg Village, and soothed by readings from a French children's story, strains of classical music and simple silence.

Helen died this afternoon, calm and at peace.

I remember how many of Helen's friends would smile and shake their heads when I met them, saying, "If only you had known Helen back when..." But I am satisfied with the nine short months I've known her. What is important is that she had the pleasure of remembering and telling her tales, and I had the pleasure of listening to them.

And when she needed to focus all her energies on breathing rather than talking, she still told her tales, often without words—she told them with her eyes, her hands, her smile. Her lessons in dying were as valuable as the lessons she has taught me in living.

I can finish this story only as I began it, with Helen's own written words:

"The last part of the journey he [Estebanico, and I will add, Helen] traveled alone... all men must travel alone the end of the journey, from the chains of early slavery to the gates of heavenly freedom... As he said and I wrote it down: What is the end of a life but the story of the life itself?" ■

My thanks to Helen's "community"—Rick Tejada-Flores, Jo Sanders, Ellen Karel, Filomena Giese, the librarians at Bancroft and Berkeley libraries—for sharing their stories of Helen with me. My thanks, too, to those on the staff at Willow Tree who came to treasure Helen's presence.

WRITER'S PROFILE

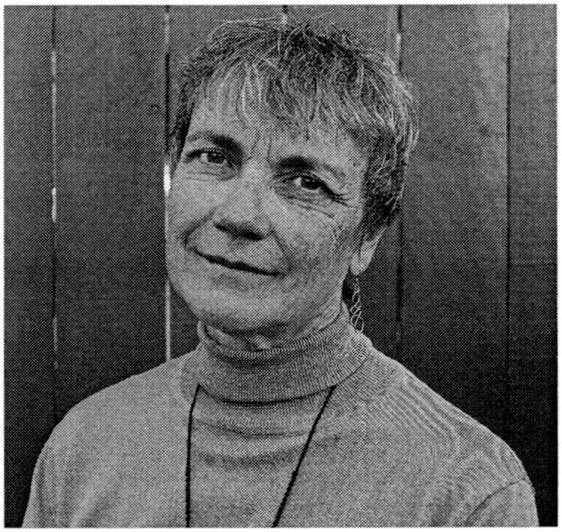

Kathleen Barrows

I never dreamed I'd get "hooked" on elders, let alone find myself signing up for workshops on Alzheimer's or reading books on aging. But that's what has happened in the last three years, ever since I fell in love with the smiles, the handholding and the wisdom that I encountered with Julia Sharp, my first *Nine Lives* elder in Volume 1. As coordinator of this second volume, I've had the good fortune of meeting every elder in this book, and my "list of elders to visit" gets longer every day. I love to laugh with them, to hear how they've encountered life's joys and challenges, and to ponder how they face their deaths.

Decades ago, when I used to visit my grandmother and great aunt in a nursing home, it was hard to relate to the white-haired wheelchair-bound seniors lining the halls. But now, at fifty-six, caring with my sister for my aging mother, I find working with elders provides invaluable lessons. It has convinced me that there is a way, even beyond words, to connect to a person's essence and that the ability to make sense of one's life in old age is an essential part of living and dying.

Most of my professional years have been dedicated to communicating across cultures, first as a researcher in bilingual education projects and later teaching English and training teachers in Brazil. Over the past ten years as a freelance writer, I've come to appreciate the importance of telling and listening to people's stories.

My remarkable friendship with Helen Rand Parish, one that Helen would call "miraculous," has taken me full circle. It brought me back to my earlier career, which was focused on Latin America, and it enabled me to look to the future, hopeful in the possibility of aging with grace, good humor and optimism, even in the face of physical frailty.

BERTY PHILLIPS

The Heritage
San Francisco, California
with
Ned Schaub

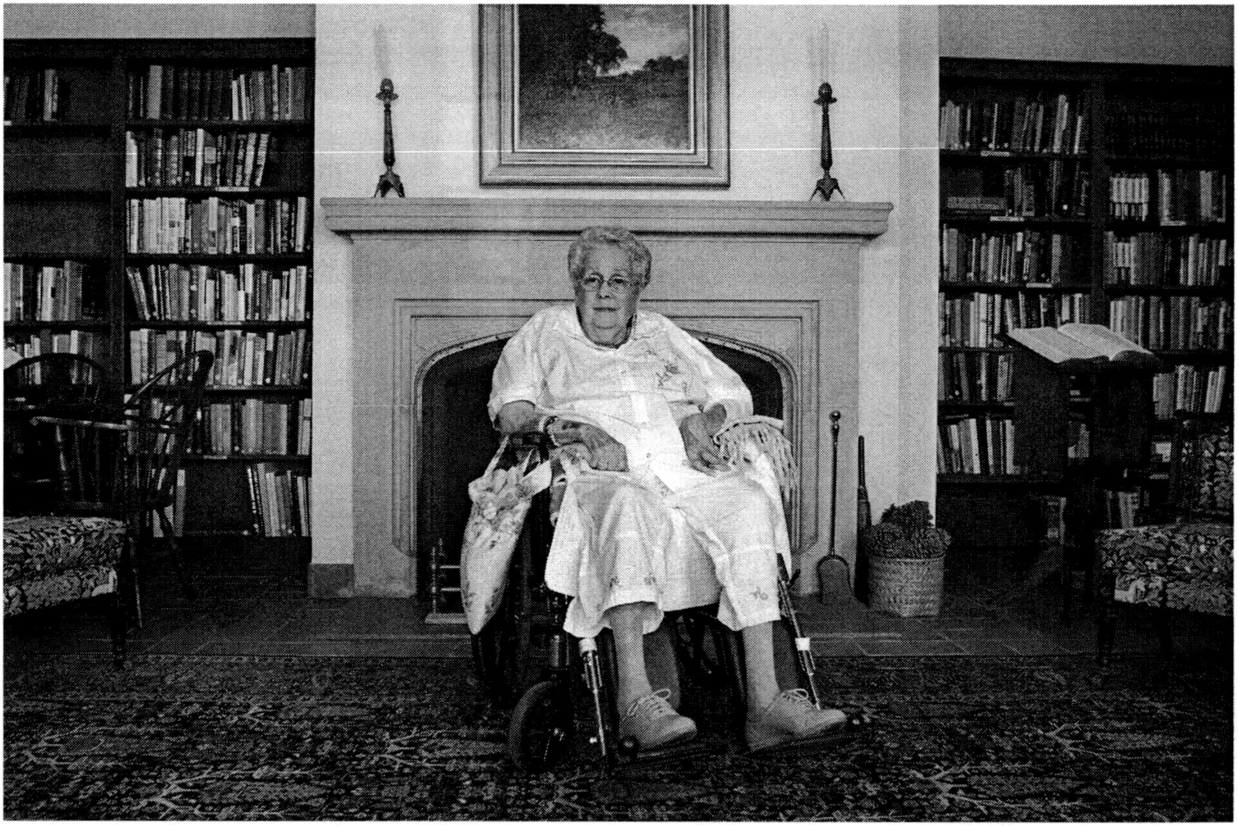

"Tell about my freedom…Tell that I was free and that it made me very happy"

Places in Time

Each of us identifies with the places where we are born, play, grow up, work, celebrate, struggle and change. To an extent, those places shape us, and we shape them and the people in them. Berty Phillips of rural Pennsylvania. Berty Phillips of suburban Los Angeles. Berty Phillips of San Francisco. Berty, like each of us, is the person that she was in each place and stage of her life, and she is Berty of this moment in time. At every place and time in her life—including this one—there has been a kind of freedom that she knew, so it is appropriate that when I asked Berty how she'd like me to tell her story she replied, "Tell about my freedom—the freedom you have when you are running free and growing up. Tell that I was free and that it made me very happy."

It seems that there are three Bertys in one person, each of them from a different place and each of them with a different story to tell.

If you ever have the opportunity to sit and listen to a person who has lived for nine decades, who is as generous with her stories and sharp as Berty Phillips, you may glimpse who that person has been at different points in time. Berty's thoughtful and descriptive stories about her life have helped me understand who she is and who she has been along the way—and how she achieved freedom in different ways at different times. Her sense of place is keen, and the qualities of those places have provided much of the fabric of her life. It seems that there are three Bertys in one person, each of them from a different place and each of them with a different story to tell.

She was very much a country girl growing up and early in her married life, and very connected to the natural landscape around her. With a big move to the West Coast, she left behind the natural surroundings she knew in rural Pennsylvania, but came to enjoy greater independence and sophistication than she had known. Arriving at The Heritage in San Francisco, almost eight years ago, she reacquainted herself with the style of smaller communities.

In a sense she has traveled a full circle, from her time in small-town and rural Pennsylvania, to the urban and suburban landscape, and back again to a small community. One day she told me, "My son John says that I came from a small town and that now I'm right back in one." The stories and thoughts that she has shared with me over the last eight months have revealed a life of significant changes and the development of her strong character. What follows is a glimpse into Berty today—and Berty along the way.

Pennsylvania and the East Coast

She was born the middle child, the only girl in a family of five children. She knows the names of wildflowers and recalls happy memories of going along with her Aunt Sue when Sue was painting. She sometimes skated down the river to school in winter. She was pestered by John Phillips—who began courting her in the sixth grade. The house where she and John were married was decorated with candles and sweet william on the window sills. They lived in a cabin just after they were married, and then with their first two children—Ann and John—in a boarding house during the war. Shortly after the family moved to East Orange, New Jersey, their third child, Frances, was born.

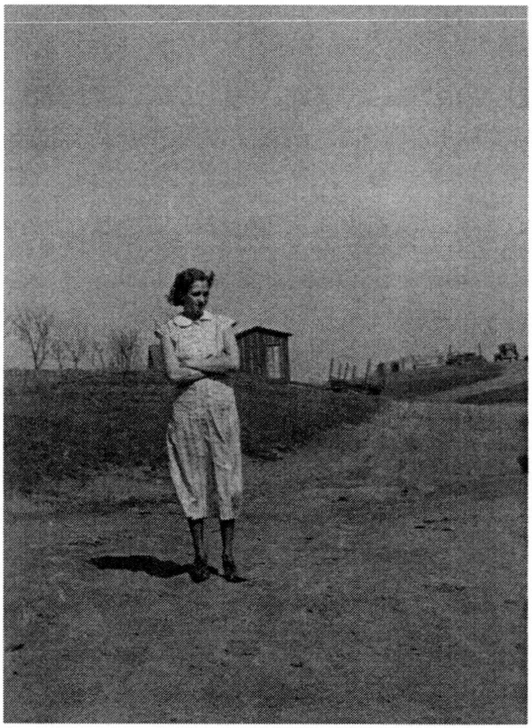

Berty in the countryside of Pennsylvania

On one wall of her room in The Heritage, there is an old color photograph that has faded to black and white. It is of a lane in rural Pennsylvania, from the county where Berty grew up. There isn't a soul to be found in the photograph and it isn't a colorful *Sunset Magazine* image. Yet it catches your eye, probably because it is black and white, very simple and a bit haunting. It's a road somewhere in another time and place, rural Pennsylvania near the home of her husband's cousin.

When I ask Berty what she'd like to see if she had the chance to go back to her original "place," she tells me "streams, woodlands and flowers." The natural surroundings of her youth seem to represent the freedom of that time, of her ability to get out in the countryside with its dense woods, low mountainous areas and small farms. Berty easily identifies each flower in the flower arrangements that decorate The Heritage and readily corrected me one day, "Not gardenia, camellia," when I had misidentified a particular blossom. And as we gaze out into The Heritage's garden one evening when I visit, she explains her feelings about Pennsylvania a bit more, "I loved the flowers that come up in the spring, the crocuses and daffodils…and the sound of rushing streams." Proud of the flora of her birth state, she giggles a bit as she considers aloud how few crocuses we see on the West Coast.

She was born in 1914 in Johnstown, which is "straight down from Pittsburgh," and the site of the historical Johnstown flood. Berty's mother grabbed a teapot out of the floodwaters that Berty's daughter Frances still has. The family moved to central Pennsylvania when she was an infant, and her father ran a coal mine and later was in the lumbering business. "Both my mother and father were very hard working, and made their kids conscious of saving. All of us helped in the garden, but we were also free and easy." She tells me that her older brothers—Elmer and Clyde—worked with their father in lumbering, her younger brother Eddie studied agriculture and her youngest brother Jimmy spent a great deal of time in the war. As she talks of her brothers, who have all died, her voice softens. "I remember that once we went to the Huntington County Fair to see my brother Elmer who had two beautiful draft horses. He had entered them in a contest and was trying to have them pull something very heavy to demonstrate their strength. He made a faint clicking sound and they just pulled it right out for him." Her feelings of affection and admiration for her brothers are obvious. Berty's brothers were very protective of her and taught her a great deal. It was they who taught her to drive, sitting by her side for hours as she grasped the steering wheel of the family auto, learning to drive on the road that led to the chicken farm that her brother Eddie eventually purchased.

"Both my mother and father were very hard working, and made their kids conscious of saving. All of us helped in the garden, but we were also free and easy."

Her stories reveal her family's love of the land they worked. Berty still recalls the variety of produce they grew in their garden—onions, tomatoes, pumpkins . . . And with talk of the land and of gardening, it seems that she has returned to her mother's kitchen. Berty describes one of her favorite recipes—coleslaw. It was made with a very thinly sliced white cabbage and a light dressing of sour cream and vinegar. It's the one thing she would love to taste most of all, she says. She then moves on to other culinary memories from her childhood: "And she made seven pies at a time…apple, pecan, pumpkin."

Berty recalls that they moved around a lot, but settled in the town of Alexandria. It was there, on the very first day of school, that she met a young man who followed her around "and didn't give up." He was John Phillips, who became her husband in November of 1937 when she was twenty-three. "We got married in my home," she recalls, "It was a small wedding. Back then there wasn't money for large weddings, and what I wanted was to be married at home. Our immediate families were there, and we were friends of the minister and his wife. This is small town stuff, and I wore a very simple, but pretty dress. We were married in front of the fireplace and there was a fire going."

Their first house was a small cottage "up at the edge of John's father's farm— with just a kitchen, a living room with a stone fireplace and one bedroom." She's happy to know from a family member who recently visited the property that her first home is still there. Speaking about good times during those days, Berty fondly remembers painting the cottage one weekend. Hard work was a part of her youth and married life – and it is integral even to the good times that she recalls.

"I always enjoyed school. I really liked geography and thinking about the different places in the world, though we didn't travel much—even when I was older." She and John were both good students. Berty went to college for a year and a half, but left it behind at the time of her marriage. John was accepted to Princeton, where his father had gone, but plans for the future were interrupted by the Depression. John went instead to RCA Radio School in Greenwich Village, New York, and ended up working at Pratt and Whitney, an airlines technology company. His job took him first to Newark, New Jersey and later to Springfield, Massachusetts.

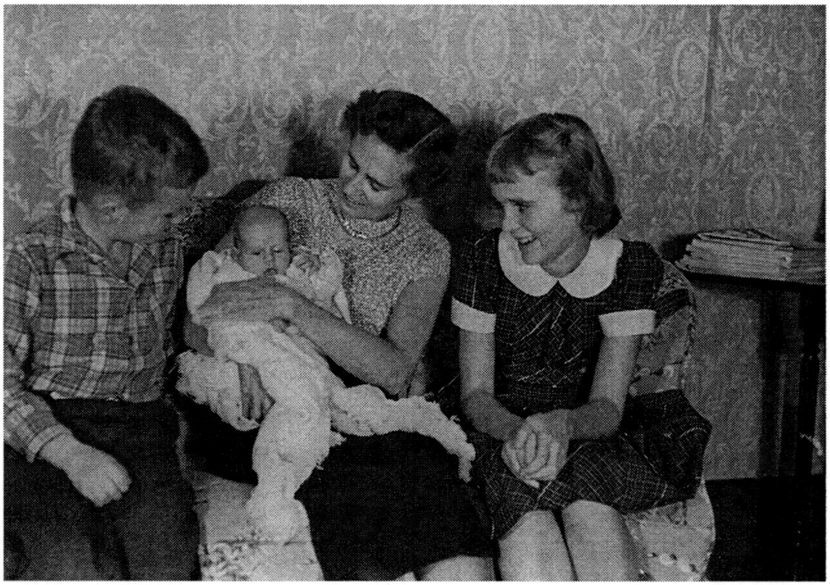

Berty with her three children

While in New Jersey, they lived in a boarding house. It was during the war and it was a difficult time for Berty. Her daughter Frances explained, "There was a severe housing shortage and she couldn't risk being kicked out of the boarding house. All of the other tenants were elderly people. She says that to avoid bothering them during the day, she kept my brother and sister out at the park all day and didn't bring them home until they were tired out and quiet. Then she did housework late into the night. When you see pictures of my family at that time, you see two skinny parents and two robust children."

The first house they owned was at 101 Longview Road in Palmer, Massachusetts —just outside of Springfield. Fran began kindergarten and Ann graduated from high school there. Fran told me, "In some ways it was a hard place to live: The town had a large Polish and large Irish population and was much divided down religious lines. My parents were 'rebels' in that they were Protestants but were best friends with Pat and Bill Donovan, who were Catholics. My father never much liked to attend church. He was put off by people who were 'officially pious,' but not kind or forgiving in their daily interactions with people. And he always liked to be doing things: sitting in church made him restless." One of the family's most famous stories about the house in Palmer, which was on a large property with a swimming pool, is about the three children sledding one winter. The pool had been drained and Ann accidentally went over the crest of a hill the wrong way and had a dramatic crash, landing in the swimming pool.

Berty was reluctant to move so far from family and the only part of the world that she had known.

While they were living in Massachusetts, John realized that he wanted to work for himself and to be at the center of the aerospace industry. For him that meant going west, so he began commuting back and forth across the country in his black 1955 T-Bird. Frances clarified, "It was actually Mother's black 1955 T-Bird, but there was a long-running family joke because when he brought it home as a new car he presented it as a gift to her even though it was obvious that he had been the one who fell for it. That car was in our family for almost twenty years." After they had moved to California, Frances drove the car in high school and her brother in college.

Los Angeles

She didn't want to leave for California, didn't want to be so far away. John was driving their T-Bird there and back, and there and back, and she finally gave in. They moved to suburban Los Angeles. Her daughter Frances recalls that she kept the house so clean it glowed. She had a Country Squire station wagon. Frances remembers her ironing in the afternoon when she got home, and that she used to call out "Ann, I mean, Fran, I mean, John." There was honeysuckle up the porch post—and passionflowers. They traveled back to the wilderness of Pennsylvania in the summers.

Berty was reluctant to move so far from family and the only part of the world that she had known. Her oldest daughter, Ann, was just beginning college in the East at the time. But Berty and the two youngest children, John and Frances, left Massachusetts for California in 1958. This signaled a time of great change for the Phillip's family, and for Berty as an individual.

John was very dedicated to his work and loved it deeply. Berty fully supported him through his long working hours. His efforts paid off and he was able to buy into the aeronautical inventions company in Santa Monica where he worked, and which came to manufacture aeronautical pieces he had designed. "He was a very good engineer and loved engineering since he was a kid. His work filled his life and made him happy," says Berty proudly. John played a key role in the invention of umbilical and in-flight disconnects mechanisms that separate space rockets from their launching pads and the stages on the rockets after they are launched. These inventions landed the company lucrative contracts with Northrop, Grumman, and Boeing. It was an exciting time for the Phillips family, and they became affluent in a way that they had never been before.

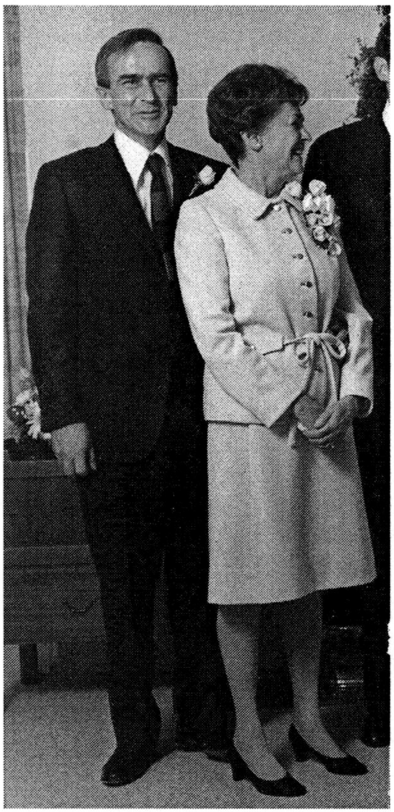
John and Berty

The young girl from Pennsylvania, who loved the simple pleasures of rural Pennsylvania life, also probably never could have imagined her husband's instrumental role in American exploration in space. John's inventions helped send America's first flight to the moon. But it wasn't without sacrifice. While John spent time in New Mexico participating in testing and traveled to Cape Canaveral for launchings, Berty took care of the family in Los Angeles. "I can still remember that evening [of the moon landing]," she says. "We were in the family room and there was a man on the moon." She pauses for a moment and then adds, "You have to do something that your heart desires. You have to stay with it, you don't stop; it's there and you're going to do it."

Frances, Berty's daughter, explains that her mother kept their home in Rolling Hills, California with great care. She laughs when she recalls the comment of the woman who bought the family home: "The oven in this house must not have ever been used." It personified her mother's skills in keeping an immaculate house, even down to the kitchen where she was constantly cooking. Her mother was an excellent cook, says Frances, and much like her mother's mother, a fantastic pie-baker. Frances tells me, "Apple was the standard, and 'Peach Supreme' was a family favorite—she made more fruit than custard, and also made homemade ice cream." During that period, Berty enjoyed her home and the simple pleasures of suburban Southern California living: shopping at the Farmers Market in Los Angeles and at the shops in Long Beach, having friends over for cocktails, going out to dinner and taking long walks in the evening.

"He was a very good engineer and loved engineering since he was a kid. His work filled his life and made him happy," says Berty proudly.

Her neighbors also made lasting impressions on her and her family. She easily recalls the vibrant personalities of friends and neighbors who led lives that seemed so far from her Pennsylvania upbringing. For example, Babe DuPont (whose real name was Gertrude) had been a professional dancer before a DuPont "threw a diamond at her." Frances recalls that her mother and the outgoing Babe bonded because they were both "East Coasters."

Her neighbor Lulu Epstein had moved to Rolling Hills from Beverly Hills with her husband George, and Berty describes her as elegant and exotically sophisticated. Lulu's young daughter complimented Berty's flower-arranging ability. She remembers the exact words, saying Berty had "a knack with flower arranging—making a few weeds into something beautiful." Still another Rolling Hills neighbor, Betty Barnes, was the only close friend that Berty had known who had been divorced. She was very independent, volunteered at UCLA's Fowler Museum and took Berty with her to lectures. Under the influence of her friend, Berty became more engaged than ever before in reading the papers and casting an educated vote.

Rolling Hills brought Berty a very different life. Yet, even though she valued her new independence and lifestyle in urban and suburban America, she was drawn out in the evenings to the sky, the stars and the moon—the simple beauty of nature that she had grown up enjoying.

But in 1975 she was faced with a type of independence that challenged her like never before. That was the year her husband John died. John had suffered rheumatic fever in his youth and lived his life with a permanently damaged heart. This had led to more serious illness in the early 1970s, until his death in 1975. At that point, Berty's life took a different shape. For the first time, she was completely on her own and independent in a new way.

"She really came into her own style, making all the choices about how she'd live her life," notes Frances. Some had thought of her along the way as the "little woman in the shadow of the big man." The six-foot-tall John was ten inches taller than his small-statured wife, Berty. But more importantly, he had had a very exciting and consuming career, while she played what some might have viewed as a strong, but quiet, supporting role. In the years after his death she proved to be a business woman in her own right, investing her money and managing her own books with great precision.

Frances recalls that just after the stroke, Berty told them repeatedly that all she wanted was her freedom.

In 1986 she sold the family home, purchased a townhouse and set it up exactly the way that she wanted to. She visited a small supermarket near her house regularly, came to know people there and had a routine that she liked. Frances recalls that "she was surrounded both at the townhouse and in the surrounding community by friends of all ages." It was perhaps the first time in her entire life that she had to make all the choices. It was a challenging and exciting time for her.

San Francisco

Her nurse Billie promised that she'd "retire when Berty expired." But, Billie retired and then came back from retirement. Frances takes Berty down along the Bay for theater and up the hill to Union Street for pizza—and shopping. Berty tells, "Franny wouldn't buy the shoes unless I bought a pair, and so we agreed that we'd both get them and let her brother John worry about the bill." She notes that the dining room at The Heritage is always beautiful for Mother's Day—pink napkins and flowers on all the tables. John Killeen, the activities director, is a very caring person. The cats that visit The Heritage's patio belong to the neighbor Mrs. Hughes' daughter. She tells me one day "Those kitties are so fat that they make us girls look slim!"

The freedom of Berty's later L.A. years ended abruptly when she suffered a stroke in 1997. Paralysis on her left side robbed her of her physical independence. It was a terrible time for all the family, admits Berty. Shortly afterwards, her two children who live in San Francisco, Frances and John, brought her to live in their city. Frances recalls that just after the stroke, Berty told them repeatedly that all she wanted was her freedom.

The Heritage is a large home for elders, located in the Marina area of San Francisco, just a few blocks from the San Francisco Bay. It has both an assisted living component, where residents live independently in rooms and apartments but receive meals and some assistance; and a skilled nursing facility, which is known as the Health Center, for residents needing constant care. The front section of The Heritage's complex, which serves as a sort of living room and reception area, is a historic red-brick building that was designed by the famed architect Julia Morgan. Originally established in 1853 as the Ladies Protection and Relief Society to care for homeless women and orphans, it was turned into an attractive center for housing and permanent care for the elderly in the 1920s. It has an elegant and stately feel, with paneled rooms, high ceilings and fireplaces. It is furnished with oriental rugs and beautiful antiques and there are a grand piano and a library full of books. The atmosphere of this historical part of The Heritage seems appropriate to Berty's bearing, to her strong and proud nature.

"When Billie comes into the room the whole place comes to order. She's just like that; she doesn't even have to say anything. They all respect her and like her."

To reach Berty's room you wind your way through the Julia Morgan section and along the edge of the independent living dining room and common areas. The Health Center, where Berty's room is located, has a more institutional feel, but is decorated with art and incorporates some of the residents' belongings into their rooms.

Her room—her "place" for this stage of her life—is simple, painted white with a window looking out onto a flowering hedge. She shares it with a roommate who speaks little. Berty has brought some remnants of her other places—many photographs and a tall wing-back chair. Her sense of place is still very evident. One week she was moved out of her room for one night while it was being painted "the same color of white." Berty paused as she told me the story, then glancing at me, added with her saucy sense of humor, "They should have painted it lime green." It's obvious that she sometimes wishes for a living space that is more individual and truly her own.

The Berty of today comes across as a strong woman who can be tough, but who also shows her strength in her sense of humor and the gentle way that she treats those around her. Her face is expressive and her voice and laugh a bit gravelly. She giggles often and is sassy. Because of the way she expresses herself, her character comes shining through—though her left side is paralyzed and she cannot walk.

Her arrival at The Heritage was not easy, but the friendship she developed with one particular nurse has made the adaptation to her new home easier. That nurse was Billie. Billie was the one who took her under her care, understood her particular needs, made her laugh, and even teased her—and it is clear that Berty has deep admiration for her. "When Billie comes into the room the whole place comes to order. She's just like that; she doesn't even have to say anything. They all respect her and like her." Billie had told Berty that she'd "retire when you expire." They were comforting words; however, shortly after Berty celebrated her ninetieth birthday, Billie retired...but only briefly.

"This experience made me grow as a human being. Though these people are not your family, you have to be truthful with them."

Berty persisted, convincing The Heritage staff, her children, and eventually and most importantly Billie that the faithful nurse and friend needed to come back. "She didn't like retirement," explains Berty, "and she said to me that she wished she could get work, just a couple of days a week." Now Billie comes on Tuesdays and Thursdays just to take care of Berty. It has meant a great deal to Berty to be able to count on one of her dearest friends coming around again. Affectionate teasing lies at the heart of their relationship. "We just have fun. There isn't anything I can count on being teased about; she'll just get me when they come up," Berty says.

Berty is very aware and considerate of those around her. On one of my visits, when one of the nurses brought her roommate back to the room early one evening to prepare her for bed, Berty commented several times, "You'll have to tell us if we are in the way."

Berty realizes that she has grown from her experience at The Heritage: "When I came here to live, I'd never lived anywhere except my individual homes. I had to learn something new. Because I was taught to be honest and fair, I knew that I had to learn to really live with other people. This experience made me grow as a human being. Though these people are not your family, you have to be truthful with them." She admits, "I was sad when I got here, but I was greeted with caring. The people here are very nice—and that makes the difference. Sometimes in the morning when I'm very tired, they're working with me and I wish they'd leave me alone. Then I think of the people in Laguna Honda Hospital—each with their own little curtained space. You know, it must be awfully hard to live like that. I count my blessings."

With her endearing personality and quick mind, Berty has made strong connections with several residents of the Health Center also. One was a pioneering woman British Air Force pilot in World War II, and there was a poet who had lived in Colorado. Another was a lesbian woman who had originally moved to San Francisco to hide from her family and then had opened up one of the city's very successful Castro district bed and breakfast establishments. But most of the residents in the Health Center suffer from dementia, and a number of them do not communicate at all. Berty wishes she could be around more young people because of their vibrancy and the quality of the conversation that she has with them.

Her sense of humor is one of the things that have carried her across the years, both now and in the past. As the process of our friendship has grown, her humor has become a part of our conversations. She knows me well enough to tease me now. Some months into our time together, Berty was in the middle of telling me a story that involved her daughter Frances. She stopped, looked at me with a mischievous expression, and said, "I guess you know who Fran is by now." Another February evening when she was fighting off a cold, she asked me to move the wastebasket closer so that she could "shoot baskets" with her used Kleenex. When I did, she said, "That's a good boy!" and giggled her gravelly laugh. When I promised her that I was being careful about not revealing private information in her story, and that there wasn't any scandalous information to include anyway, she commented, "Well, I guess that I'll have to make something up."

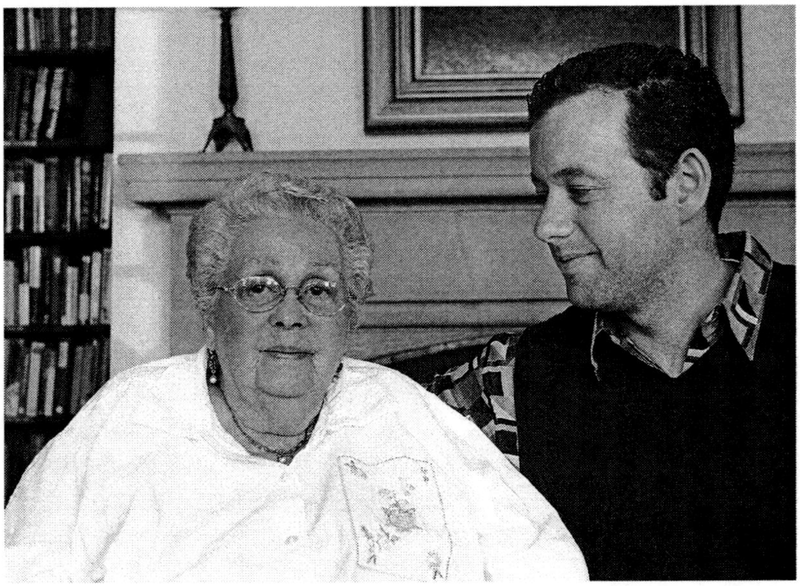

Berty with her writer, Ned

Her family, too, appreciates her wry humor, and what Frances describes as her "self-deprecating little quips" which are "quick," with "her timing right on the mark." Both Berty and Frances have told me the story about their Rolling Hills neighbor girl's comment concerning Berty's flower arrangements. Because of the way this compliment was revealed to Berty, a playful family rule came to exist. The rule dictates that if someone hears a compliment about another family member, he or she will only reveal it if someone else in the family gives them a compliment first.

Berty delights in the time that both Frances and John spend with her every week, visiting her and taking her on adventures in the nearby neighborhoods. She seems almost giddy with excitement when they arrive. She recently mentioned, "When we went out on Mother's Day, Fran pushed me along to the restaurant in the rain, and then when we came out it had stopped." There was an interesting mix of pleasure and defiance in this little story.

"My three kids turned out well...They are good people, very decent—and they were prepared to be grown-ups."

At almost ninety-one, Berty awaits the arrival of another great-grandchild, and keeps track of when her four granddaughters, three great-grandchildren, and her daughter Ann (who lives on the East Coast) will be coming through town. Her family is the indicator of her success—they represent her life's work, and much of her peace comes from enjoying their company and from knowing how they live their lives. "My three kids turned out well," she says to me. Wondering if she were referring to their jobs or families, I asked her what she meant. "They are good people, very decent—and they were prepared to be grown-ups," she responded. "They give me credit for being their mother."

She recounts a nice visit she recently had with both John and Frances, "It was raining and John had brought a picnic, so he said, 'Let's just go to the Cedar Room down the hall to have our lunch.'" She gazed peacefully out the window, confident in her accomplishment of having raised a good family, and said, "They had such a good time talking. It's so nice when your kids like one another—and they had so much to talk about that we just had a very good time. Things fall in line when you're with your family. You talk about this and that, and it goes on and on."

Berty's family traditions continue to be handed down through the family. Now, at Thanksgiving, it's Frances who makes the pies—like Berty did in Southern California and Berty's mother did in Pennsylvania. Frances has also taken on the baking of the family's traditional Christmas cookies that her mother always used to make. Though her sense of taste has suffered some with her stroke, Berty can tell whether the recipe is on the mark or not. "You've got just the right amount of almond extract, Fran," she'll comment after testing one of her daughter's creations.

Twilight and Freedom

Sometimes Berty gets frustrated with her situation or with the way something is handled at The Heritage. Sometimes she is sad. One day she mentions that she had observed some fellow residents dancing and was overcome with the full realization that she would never dance—or even walk—again. But it's her predominant characteristics that I have observed over the months that shine through—her strong will, quick wit and timing, gentleness, sweetness, shyness, down-to-earth nature, courage in the face of discomfort and inconvenience, patience, acceptance and her strong sense of privacy.

Her physical limitations do not limit the strength of her character, her appreciation of the world around her, her connection to individuals or her sense of adventure.

She is forever a careful observer of nature around her, noticing the flowers outside in the garden and those inside, cut and arranged by the woman who lives in The Heritage's caretaker cottage. She frequently comments about a specific flower, describing what she likes most about it.

Like many of the residents, she's also fascinated by and affectionate toward The cats, Joey and Lucky, that hang around in the garden seeking the attention of doting Heritage cat lovers. She talks very sweetly to them or about them, "Joey needs to go home and get his dinner," and then when Joey sits up proudly she imagines his voice, "He says, 'Do you like this pose better?'"

Though it's hard for me to understand how one deals with the loss of physical capacity and all that it entails, I can't stop thinking that Berty has mastered the current situation of her life, as she has done in every other stage of her life. In doing so she has achieved freedom once again. Her physical limitations do not limit the strength of her character, her appreciation of the world around her, her connection to individuals or her sense of adventure. Her resilience shines through in a remark she made to her daughter: "I said to Fran, 'I'm the only one of my siblings left, I suppose that means I should do something worthwhile,' and Fran said that I should, and I said, 'Well, I'm not going to!'" With a chuckle and a glimmer in her eye she also tells me the story about a harmless, but slightly abrasive exchange with one of the nurses: "I didn't give in. When I'm in a fight I win."

It seems that just about every other week Berty tells me that Frances has once again rolled her in her wheelchair up the hill to Union Street for pizza. "I told Fran, 'You know, I'm hungry for pizza,' and she said 'Do you mind if I push you up to Union Street?'" Berty—the one from rural

Pennsylvania who enjoyed the sounds of rushing streams and the native flowers; the one from Los Angeles, who tried to spot the stars beyond the L.A. skyline on evening walks; and now the one from The Heritage—still likes to get out to see the moon over the bay. Her body has changed in ways that limit her physically, but her mind is strong, her spirit full of fire and her country-girl nature alive and well. There is a kind of freedom in these things that is very powerful—perhaps more powerful than any other freedom that she has known. ■

A Note of Thanks: Many thanks to Berty for the wonderful adventure I am having in getting to know her. I also thank her daughter Frances for spending time with me in conversation; for supplying me with family photos and a video; and for letting me borrow some of the lines (listed in the italicized paragraphs) from a tribute prepared for her mother's ninetieth birthday.

WRITER'S PROFILE

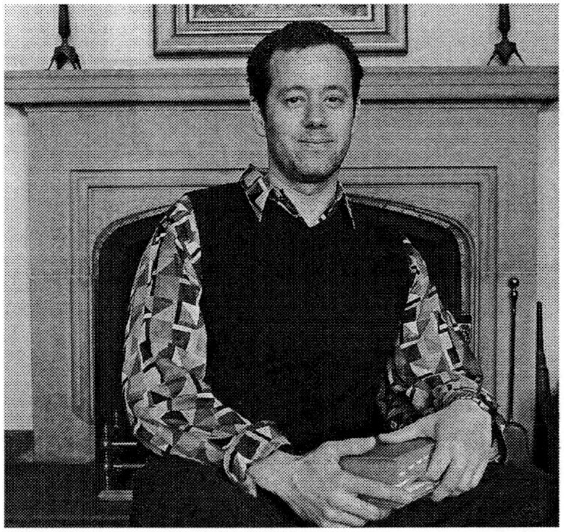

Ned Schaub

I am a Chicago native, but lived in Springfield, Illinois for much of my youth and spent time in the summer and during holidays in the small Southern Illinois town of Olney. My parents both came from Olney and my heritage is there. My great-grandparents on my mother's side of the family had sixteen children, and I grew up in the company of many cousins and elders. The experiences of knowing them, loving them, and learning from them are at the core of my life.

Getting to know Berty reminds me of Olney and family, and it is one of my greatest San Francisco experiences. In quiet evening discussions, Berty and I share thoughts on everything from the mysteries of our lives to thoughts about the flowers around us. She has given me some important advice about the need to slow down, and even poked fun at the pace I keep. I realize that as we take time to laugh together and silently observe the cats in the garden, I have ended up following her advice. Berty has become a great mentor and friend.

I am currently working on my master's degree in nonprofit management, and my graduate thesis will focus on the delivery of hospice and palliative care in the Bay Area and what private funding could do to improve it. I began my career working in Chicago nonprofit organizations that serve youth, elders, and immigrant populations. I came to San Francisco in May of 2001 to join the Gordon and Betty Moore Foundation, where I have served as a program officer making grants in the fields of eldercare and environmental conservation. Prior to that, I worked for the MacArthur Foundation's environment program. I received a BA in writing from Knox College in Galesburg, Illinois.

TAKESHIRO SAKAI

Laguna Honda Hospital
San Francisco, California
with
Lisa Ko

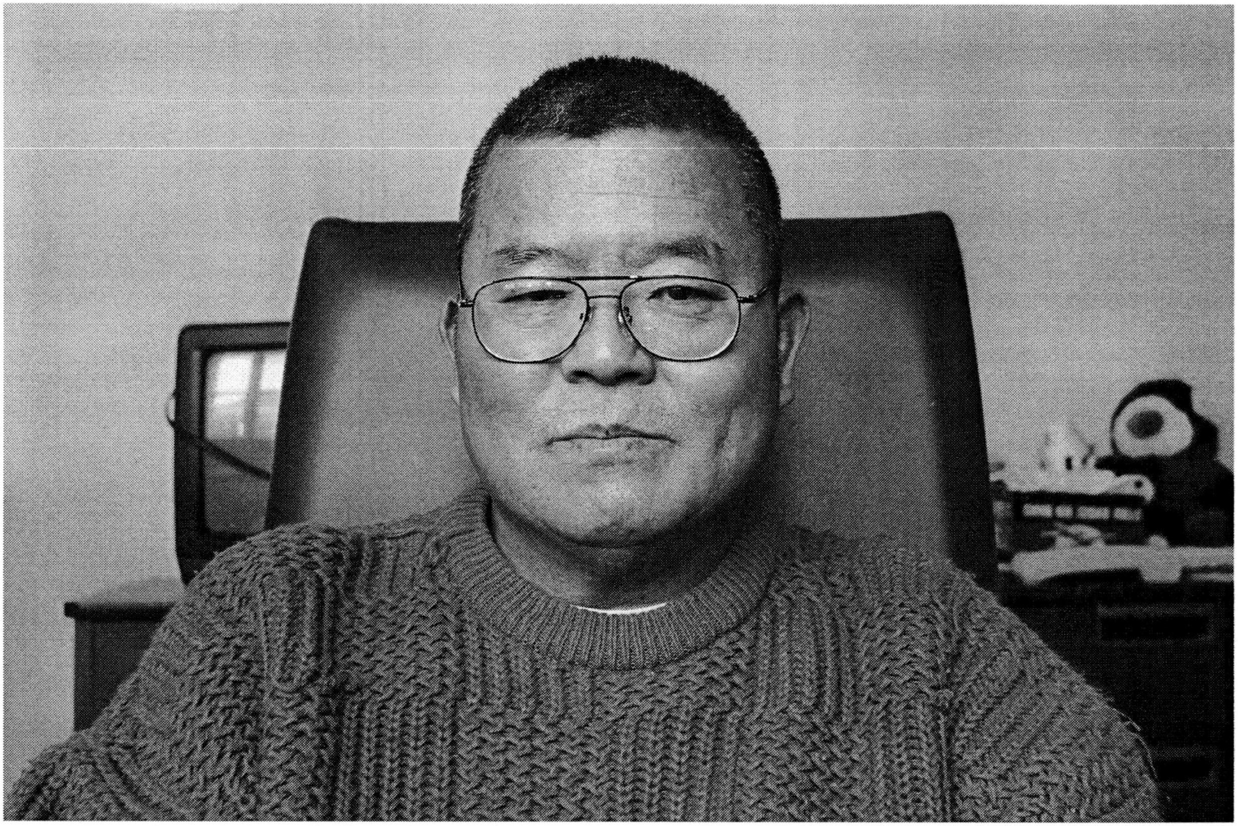

"My story is a sad story"

The first time we meet, Takeshiro Sakai tells me that his life has been a sad one.

"My story is a sad story," he says. "I should not be here." He looks around at the barren walls of his room. Besides his wife, who is only able to visit him once a week, I am his only visitor.

The youngest of the elders in this volume, Takeshiro, who goes by the nickname Take [pronounced tah-kee], isn't even officially a senior citizen yet. When I first meet him in August 2004, he is only sixty-three and looks even younger with his salt-and-pepper hair cropped close to his head and his face relatively unlined. Yet Take moves slowly, always wearing his requisite thick glasses, black watch, and yellow plastic hospital wristband. He shuffles down the halls of San Francisco's Laguna Honda Hospital, where he has lived since he suffered a massive stroke at the age of sixty. No longer able to work or live on his own, he was forced to sell his beloved restaurant and leave the Alameda home he shared with his wife, Eiko, for San Francisco's only public nursing facility.

Take's English is halting at best. As we talk, I find myself conversing in slightly broken English, as I do with some of my older relatives. We agree to meet every Tuesday night after I get off from work.

When I arrive at Laguna Honda for my second visit, Take is waiting for me in the lobby, dressed in blue pajamas and flip-flops. As I walk towards him I realize he has dozed off in one of the overstuffed chairs. I call his name, and he looks up, surprised that he has a visitor and glad to see me.

I call his name, and he looks up, surprised that he has a visitor and glad to see me.

Take and I talk in the library of Laguna Honda's Clarendon Hall, where he also takes his art classes. He is in the ELDERGIVERS' Art With Elders program at the hospital, taking weekly painting classes. Since his stroke made hobbies such as cooking and fishing impossible, painting has become one of his favorite activities. Paintings by the Art With Elders students line the walls of the library, and Take proudly shows me some of his work, including a picture of a dense forest dotted with bright yellows, greens and reds.

"Has your wife taken you out lately?" I ask.

Take nods. "Yes, to the art exhibition." Some of his paintings were part of an Art With Elders show at the Rincon Center in downtown San Francisco. "She [my wife] liked my paintings and wants to buy them."

By the time Take finishes drawing, he's forgotten why he brought the word up in the first place.

"Was she born in Japan, too?" Take nods. "Did you meet her here?"

"Yes." Before I can get another word in, he says, "Today I want to tell you a story about Pescadero."

Despite Take's effort to change the subject, it seems there is no story about Pescadero. His monologue is rambling, unfocused. "Mr. Wong brought me there. Do you know Hearst Castle? Geoducks were small." Take is frustrated. His hands shake. He stops and starts with new topics. "Have you ever tried *matsutake*? It's a mushroom... a Japanese mushroom, very expensive, an import. You slice it and eat over rice. I used to cook it in my restaurant. Very good."

I try to lead him back on track, but I don't know what questions will spur the story because I don't know what the story is supposed to be about.

"When did you sell your restaurant?" I ask.

Take looks confused. He has been talking to me in Japanese, forgetting that I don't understand it. "2090... no, 2000, no, I don't know what you are saying."

"2001," I say. "A few years ago?"

"This is 2004 right now?"

"Yes, now it is 2004. But soon it will be 2005."

"2005." Take shakes his head. "What did I do in 2004? Nothing. What am I doing? I am wasting time."

I try to cheer him up. "You were in an art show in 2004. And in 2005 you will be in a book!" But we both know it is a weak attempt. What is there for Take to look forward to? As he told me in our first conversation, he doesn't want to be here.

Talking with Take can be difficult. English is his second language, and although he has lived in the U.S. for more than three decades, his numerous health problems have diminished his fluency. Conversation is excruciatingly slow as he searches for the right words. He's frustrated easily, his mind wanders. He blurts out things in Japanese, attempts to draw for me pictorial representations of the words we can't translate. But even drawing is slow going as he struggles to grip the pen. It is painstaking. By the time Take finishes drawing, he's forgotten why he brought the word up in the first place.

Interviewing someone with diminished motor and mental skills soon proves to be a challenge for which no amount of experience in journalism has prepared me. Take himself is an unreliable narrator. Some weeks are better than others. Sometimes he starts off with a strong thought and then loses it mid-sentence, unable to get it back. His sentences crisscross and his stories loop back on one other. I wish I knew some Japanese or even had an interpreter. Soon I realize that being patient and letting him talk isn't the solution. Take's short-term memory is too spotty, and he needs me to prod his stories along and tell him if I've already heard him tell me something before.

Sometimes he starts off with a strong thought and then loses it mid-sentence, unable to get it back. His sentences crisscross and his stories loop back on one other.

After we talk for an hour, I tell Take I have to leave, and that I'll be back next week. He looks surprised. "Oh... only an hour?" I decide to stay and talk with him a while longer. "I had the restaurant and then the surgery," he says, referring to his career as a San Francisco restaurant owner. "I had heart problems... blood problems... I should not be here right now. So many surgeries, so much with the surgeon."

I ask Take where he had surgery. "Brain," he says, pointing to his head. The back of his head is flattened slightly, and a series of thick scars provide evidence of past brain surgeries. But he goes on to enumerate his other surgeries. "Nose," he says, pointing to his ears. "Ears?" I ask, trying to clarify. "No," he responds, but then switches his answer to "yes" and adds, "I have heart transplant." I tell him there is someone that must be looking out for him, and he is lucky to have good doctors helping him. "I don't want to be here," he says. "But I guess I was meant to be here."

When I leave, Take sees me to the door. "Thank you," he says.

"No, thank you," I tell him. "For telling me your stories. I'll see you next week at the same time."

"Are you taking the bus home?" he asks, concerned. It's dark out and cold.

I tell him it's no problem, the ride back to my house is a quick one.

He thinks about this for a moment and agrees. "Okay, Lisa, good night."

When I visit Take in Clarendon Hall, I simply walk in through the back entrance. No one ever asks me what I am doing here or if I need help, although in the coming months I will begin to recognize the residents that stand outside in the early evening smoking their post-dinner cigarettes. Laguna Honda's size and institutional feel are markedly different from the few nursing facilities I have visited before: a private nursing home that I

Take's shelves contain a stack of art supplies: a can of paintbrushes, watercolor paper from a local art store.

volunteered in during high school, another more costly facility where my aunt worked as a dietician.

Established in 1866 as a home for the city's poor, Laguna Honda sits atop a hill in the quiet, foggy neighborhood of Forest Hills, housing nearly 1,200 patients in its multiple buildings. Some of the structures date back to the early 1900s and are undergoing extensive renovation. It is the largest nursing home in the U.S. To reach Laguna Honda, I walk from the nearby subway station up the hill's steep and crumbling stairs, then along a winding path past dirt pits, trailers, darkened Port-A-Potties, and yellow tape marking the construction sites that are perpetually under progress. Some nights, the fog is so thick I can barely see the steps in front of me.

Take lives on the third floor of Laguna Honda's Clarendon Hall, which is home to 160 people, many of them like Take, requiring long-term assisted living and nursing care. A quarter of the hospital's population is Asian, as is nearly three-fourths of the staff. Take's room is the back room of a two-room double. The front room is home to his roommate, who is sitting on the edge of his bed, watching television and eating his dinner silently when I arrive. Both men's rooms are just large enough for a bed, a lamp, a small bookshelf, a nightstand and a table with a small television. Take's shelves contain a stack of art supplies: a can of paintbrushes, watercolor paper from a local art store.

On my way to the door, I pass a recreation room where a few residents sit, some in wheelchairs, watching a blaring TV. Outside, men and women in their thirties chain-smoke on benches in the courtyard. In recent years, the hospital has been a site of controversy in San Francisco politics. A lack of funding and space forced it to accept younger psychiatric patients, some with violent tendencies, into its traditionally eldercare facilities. But residents always stop and chat with me as I sit in the lobby and wait for Take, even if it's just to make banal conversation about the weather with a stranger.

As I walk to the subway station from Laguna Honda, I think about my own parents, who are the same age as Take. They had visited me the prior week en route from their home in New Jersey to a trip to Australia, New Zealand and Fiji. My parents are both retired and finally traveling the world after decades of working and saving money. During their visit, we took walks around Golden Gate Park, where my father, a former runner who was born a year before Take, looked at the high school track teams jogging around Stow Lake and lamented not being able to run like he used to. Yet a week later he would be trekking through the streets of Sydney and Melbourne, practicing his ballroom dancing skills in local dance clubs. We also met with my great-aunt and uncle, in their eighties and living in San Francisco's Sunset District, where they spend their days socializing with friends in the neighborhood and taking walks to nearby Ocean Beach. We all agreed that San Francisco is a good place for senior citizens and retirees, and I hope that my parents and I myself will have the same quality of life in our later years.

For Take, his immigrant story started with many similarities to my own family's story. Like Take, my parents arrived in America from Asia—the Philippines—in their mid-20s, both college graduates who proceeded to work hard at multiple jobs and save up enough money to purchase their own home. Both my mother and father ended up in New York City, where they met, married and helped sponsor other family members to come to North America. Take himself obtained a green card and eventually attained the dual middle-class success stories of being both a business owner and a homeowner. In every aspect it could have—should have—been the fulfillment of the American Dream. Take married a fellow Japanese immigrant. They worked together at a restaurant that they owned, bought property, did well. But instead of retiring together, Take is living out the rest of his life in a public hospital, walking and talking at the speed of someone twenty years his senior—this at a time when he should be starting his retirement, perhaps using these years for travel.

For Take, his immigrant story started with many similarities to my own family's story.

Take was born in Nagoya, Japan, on July 9, 1941. In 1944, his family moved to Nagano, a larger industrial city in Japan he describes as a "military city." It was World War II. Some of Take's earliest memories are of the war. "Do you remember when America bombed Japan?" I ask, referring to the atomic bombing and destruction of Hiroshima and Nagasaki in 1945.

"Yes," he says. "Yes, the bombing. When I was four, the Americans occupied Japan. Japan was losing the war. My father did not fight. We thought Japan would never win the war, not over the U.S. People in Japan were giving away cooking metals to the government so they could melt it down for war materials. There was a power difference. Japan never expect to win against such a big country."

"My family was from Hokkaido," Take tells me. Hokkaido is an island in northernmost Japan. "It's snowy there. I have two brothers and one sister, all ten or more years older than me. I am the youngest. My sister always looked young, like my mother. No gray hairs. My mother died when I was in high school. She was young. But by the time I was in high school, my mother no more."

"I always like art, but I don't believe I have ability to be an artist. I would like to paint instead, do whatever."

Take's siblings were born in Hokkaido, but the family moved to Nagoya before he was born. In Hokkaido, he says, his parents tried to grow rice, but they found gold instead. "And gold was better than rice! My mother saved gold every day, every little bit, and traded it for money. But there was no work in Hokkaido. The fields are abandoned, the farmers had to leave. So they moved to Nagoya."

In Nagoya, Take's father had to find work. "My father was a professional military man," he explains. "He went to military school, but then he was wounded. He got shot with a machine gun in his thigh. It was very painful. So he retired. He went to shrine school and studied the Shinto religion. He studied the *kendo* sword and made it to fourth level, a high level not so many people get." Take himself also studied martial arts at Chuo University and even taught judo classes for two years at the University of California in San Francisco.

At Chuo, Take studied commercial law, a fact that surprised me because of his career as a restaurant owner and entrepreneur, and his continuing interest in art. "So you wanted to become a lawyer?" I asked.

He pauses and laughs "No, no... no lawyer. But I studied business law. It was an easy choice, I could get admission. But I never want to be lawyer. I regret my mistake. Regret beginning to study law. I always like art, but I don't believe I have ability to be an artist. I would like to paint instead, do whatever."

During college he worked at a gas station in Osaka, Japan's second largest city. He also spent one summer driving a truck in Hokkaido. But out of all the children in his family, Take was the only one to leave Japan. After he got to the U.S., his father remarried and eventually passed away.

"I don't know what happened to our house in Nagano now, after my father died," Take explains. "They sold it. It had so much history. So many generations lived there. Many ancestors. There was a village and a family graveyard around a temple. Many Sakais were in that graveyard—some killed by war. The village had three temples and my family owned one."

Today, Take's siblings are all married. His sister lives in the mountain region of Niigata, where she and one of his brothers had attended university. As the youngest, Take often felt left out of his older siblings' lives. "They were very close," he says. "Sometimes when I was younger I envied them. They cooperated together, even when they were very young."

It's clear that Take feels like the black sheep of his family. "My family was very good until not long ago," he says. "I was the worst. I don't have success. I play around too much. One of my brothers is president of a small electric company. His son is also a graduate of Waseda University, very good school. Another brother graduate from Niigata." Take hasn't seen his family for decades, ever since he left Japan. He only keeps in minimal touch with his siblings. "My family doesn't know I had surgery. They don't know I live here in Laguna Honda. Our relation is no good. Only once a year I call them, on New Year's. They still think I live in Alameda with my wife. I don't want them to know that she is alone."

"My family was very good until not long ago," he says. "I was the worst. I don't have success. I play around too much."

Take and I usually meet after he eats dinner, when most of the Clarendon Hall residents are glued in front of the television set in the large rec room, picking food off their plates or playing trivia games led by an enthusiastic employee. There is always someone using the building's sole computer in the library, a young Asian American man browsing online news, while an older white man in a wheelchair reads the daily papers at the table next to us.

I start to think that perhaps the computer could be a way for Take to get in touch with his estranged family. Most likely, his brother would have e-mail at his company. Or if Take weren't interested in corresponding with family or old friends, he could use the computer's Internet connection to read websites, such as online news sites. I ask him if he has ever used a computer before, and he says no and immediately asks, "Can you teach me computer?" Each week after that, he reminds me. "Next week... computer." When the computer is finally free one evening, I try to teach him how to turn it on and point and click with the mouse. But it turns out to be a far more daunting task than I had imagined. Take's lack of motor skills and hand-eye coordination make handling a mouse and keyboard difficult, and attempting to teach someone how to browse the Internet—something he has never heard of—requires a dismantling of all my technological assumptions. But I still keep wishing that there could be some way to get Take back in touch with his old friends.

I [Lisa] moved far from my home and family to a place I had never been before and where I knew no one, for many of the same reasons that Take did—adventure, novelty, escape.

Take came to the United States on an ocean liner in 1968, when he was twenty-six years old. His journey took two weeks. It was not unlike my own move out to San Francisco from New York City when I was twenty-six years old. I moved far from my home and family to a place I had never been before and where I knew no one, for many of the same reasons that Take did—adventure, novelty, escape. Instead of traveling by boat, I flew on a red-eye flight, with two suitcases stashed in the overhead compartment. Like Take, I had never planned on staying in California for so long.

When he arrived in the U.S., Take first lived in Los Angeles, where he worked a series of jobs through the under-the-table arrangements of the Japanese immigrant community. These communities are everywhere across the U.S., a common way for recent immigrants to establish a foothold into the community, regardless of their visa status. As a young man, Take's rebellious streak often got him in trouble with his employers. "In L.A. I worked for one Japanese restaurant for a while but I got fired," he explains. "I was absent, not show up. No responsibility! Then I found a job in San Francisco, so I had to move. I came here and worked as a gardener a few days. Then in a San Francisco restaurant, but I got fired again. The chef was strict and I was late. It was easy to fire me, with no visa. But I wanted to whale."

Whaling is the first thing that Take talks to me about when we meet. Not a week goes by that he doesn't mention it. Even when I was first introduced to Take, he announced, "Did you know I worked on a whaling ship?"

It takes many visits for me to piece together the puzzle. The ship was actually a boat with a crew of five men, and Take worked on it for one month. It was docked under the Golden Gate Bridge in the Pacific Ocean off the shores of San Francisco, where the whales passed as they migrated down the coast from Alaska during the winter months. The workers on the ship tried to kill two whales a day using harpoons. One of Take's former restaurant co-workers was the ship's captain—ranked number two in whaling in the region, Take said. He worked on the boat with his friend Bun, who also went for the experience and adventure.

Experience and adventure—even decades later, living housebound at

Laguna Honda, these themes remain important to Take. "It was a good experience, right?" I ask him and he agrees. "Not many people can say that they worked on a whaling boat."

"Have you ever tasted whale?" Take asks.

I shake my head.

"It tastes like meat. You can put lots of salt on it."

Take hands me an Art With Elders calendar, which features the artwork of elders living in San Francisco Bay Area nursing homes. The month of January features Take with his artwork and a brief biography. He shows me the painting—a stormy swirl of browns, purples and dark blues—that was exhibited at the art show at the Rincon Center. It depicts a view of two large whales as seen from above, swimming in an ocean highlighted by flecks of orange and red. A smaller baby whale swims in between, surrounded and protected by the two larger whales.

"This story I told you," Take says. I read the text in the calendar. It was a story he had tried to tell me the first week we met. Take had been working on the whaling boat, trying to kill two whales a day. He drew a picture of a harpoon in my notebook to illustrate this, explaining that it took three or four hours for a whale to die. After the whalers speared the whale, they had to drag it out of the water while it was dying, but still breathing a little. "It was hard to think of eating at that time because I was sad," he says. "Because the whale was dying."

Whales often migrate in pairs, or even groups or families. While on the ship, Take saw what he called "husband and wife whales" swimming together with their children, mindless of the harpoons that awaited them. But as a whaling ship employee, it was his job to help kill these whales, breaking up the family. As he explains, it was heartbreaking to have to kill one of the parents and not the other because then the other would be left alone. Whales are attached to their partners. Even if one of the whale "spouses" were killed, the other would follow the carcass as the boat hauled it away, unable to let it go. It was this image—of two large whales, which were caught and strapped to the sides of the boat, followed by a baby whale—that stuck with Take even thirty years later, when he replicated it in his painting. The ship was dragging the parents of the baby whale into the bay. Take had never seen such a sad thing before. As the calendar's description of his painting explains, it was at that moment that Take decided that he would never again

While on the ship, Take saw what he called "husband and wife whales" swimming together with their children, mindless of the harpoons that awaited them.

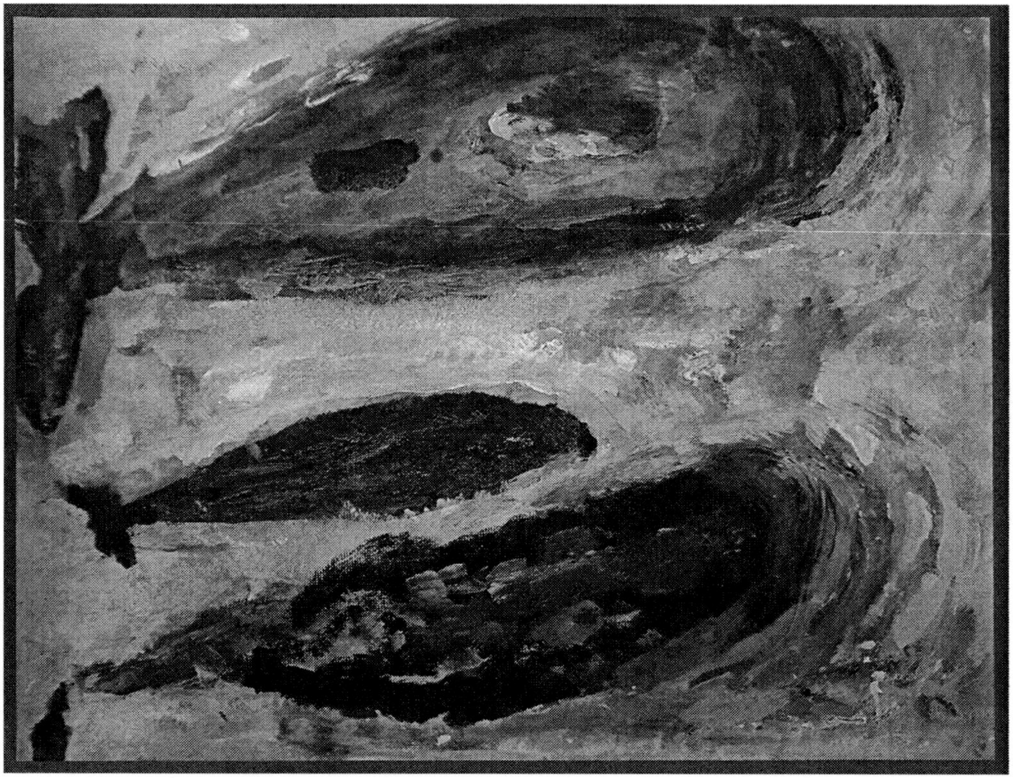

Takeshiro's painting of the whale family

hunt these great sea mammals.

"Those were hard times," he tells me. We stop talking so he can wipe the tears from his eyes.

As the months pass, I start to get frustrated when Take insists on talking more about whales. Although the time he spent on the whaling boat composed but a tiny portion of his life, with the way he repeats the whaling stories over and over again one would think it was his entire career. We might be talking about his childhood or his work at the restaurant, and mid-sentence, Take will stop talking, turn a conversational 180, and begin to talk about whales. "They struggle but not for too long. The harpoon... the spear... it's about five inches thick, no, fifteen inches long..." He ruminates again and again on whether or not whales have feelings like humans, unable to fully forget his implication in helping to kill these majestic animals.

"Whale society and human society is same. Same crazy. Whales are animals, us animals too."

"Are they sympathetic?" he asks. "Do they feel, like humans?" He returns repeatedly to the story of the family of whales, the pain of one whale at seeing its partner killed. Even Take's ship captain had said he hated to see this scene, even if he had seen it many times before.

"Why are whales your favorite subject?" I ask Take one night. "Why do you keep talking about them?" We are swapping anecdotes, good-naturedly complaining about "people who make you crazy."

He sits and thinks. "Whale society and human society is same. Same crazy. Whales are animals, us animals too. When one whale is dying, strapped to a boat, the other child or husband or wife approaches and says 'Are you okay?' The other one says, 'No, I am not okay. I am dying. This boat is making me crazy.'"

On one of our weekly visits, Take is wearing dress slacks and a neat sweater in lieu of his usual sweatpants, fleece pullover jacket and slippers. He tells me that his wife had come to visit him today. They had gone out for dinner at a Chinese restaurant in San Francisco's Inner Richmond neighborhood. Eiko still lives in the couple's house in Alameda, an island in the San Francisco Bay. She works six days a week as a housecleaner and on Mondays, her one day off, she visits Take, driving through a tunnel, across a bridge and into the city of San Francisco to take her husband out to dinner. She brings him presents, too, reminders of the outside world: painting supplies, videotapes of Japanese movies that he watches on the small TV set in his room.

"I came to America because I wanted to be by myself," he explains. "I wanted to be alone, no outside contact."

Take shakes his head. "My wife works six days a week. Too much work. She doesn't want to not work and not make money." He worries about her constantly, about her working too much, about her living alone in the house. One day, there is a small earthquake in the Bay Area and Take tells me he was worried about Eiko all day until she called to say she was all right. He feels guilty that he got sick and has to live away from her. He worries about the expenses, the medical bills.

"I came to America because I wanted to be by myself," he explains. "I wanted to be alone, no outside contact. But then I met my wife. We were introduced through friends about two or three years after I arrived in San Francisco. Immigration is tough. I had no visa, no money, so hard to get job. My friend introduce me to very nice lawyer. I applied for visa and I was denied. But then I married my wife. She had green card."

Like Take, his wife Eiko was a pioneer, a black sheep of sorts with a thirst for adventure. Like him, she was the only member of her family to leave Japan and come to America. They were each other's only family member on the continent.

"She was like me," Take says. "We wanted freedom. That's why we always in agreement, the same. She is the only person I trust, with business, with everything. When we met, she did hair styling in beauty salon and I was gardening. It was so long ago. We don't make baby, no second generation. Something was wrong. So there was a little loneliness. Especially there were close friends who had three kids, each one graduate college. I never had that."

I realized then how much Take must miss his wife. Our conversations are full of his stories about the many trips he and Eiko took together. They went to Seattle and hunted for mushrooms, dodging bear hunters in the woods. They drove up California's Highway 1 to Petaluma and fantasized about buying a run-down cabin that they saw in the forest and fixing it up for themselves. Take had always been an avid fisher and Eiko joined him on his fishing trips, driving out to Lake Tahoe with a group of their friends to catch some trout, or on some days not catching much at all, but just hanging out together.

Perhaps this is why the story of the whales has continued to resonate with him. One whale dying, being dragged away against its will, its partner desperately swimming beside it, unable to let go. When Take wonders what these two whale spouses must be saying to one another—"No I'm not okay. I'm dying"—he might also be thinking of his own situation of languishing in a hospital. Like the child in Take's depicted whale family, Take himself was once forced to fend for himself, alone in a strange country. And like the whale spouses, he now finds himself alone again later in life, separated from his wife against his will.

On my walk back to the subway that night, I call my mother in New Jersey to say hello and tell my parents that I love them. I walk the steps back to my apartment from the station on autopilot, forgetting how the streets of this city, which was once so foreign to me when I moved here sight unseen, were now simply second nature. Moving to another city by myself is one of the scariest and most exhilarating things I have ever done—the rush of being completely anonymous in a new place at odds with knowing nobody at all. It was the sense of being history-less, free of context, with the ability to write your own story.

"It was the '60s. There were hippies. Very happy people, the hippies. But crazy."

Despite Take's university degree, in San Francisco he worked mainly as a manual laborer. His lack of a visa and English language skills made him difficult to hire. He worked as a gardener for several years, then as a contract landscaper and construction worker, helping to build a number of homes in Alameda. He planted, poured cement and concrete. "These were new things, that I had never done before. It was hard work, heavy work. But I was a hard worker."

San Francisco in the '60s was a different time, the hippie heyday still reflected in the city's stereotype. "The first time I came to the area, I didn't know anything about Haight Ashbury," Take says. "It was the '60s. There were hippies. Very happy people, the hippies. But crazy. One time I was parking my motorcycle outside. My wife and I were not married yet but we were living together in Haight Ashbury. I drove her to work each morning in the neighborhood, in a beauty salon. But each day when I came out there was another part missing from my motorcycle. Thieves were stealing it piece by piece!" he laughs. "One day the battery was gone!"

In his thirties and forties, Take tried his hand at a number of business opportunities. He was always seeking to make his big break, but also having no shortage of adventures in the process. He chased all kinds of successful and not-so-successful moneymaking schemes up and down the West

"My friend's son started playing with the clams and the clam got angry and bit him!" We both laugh together at the comical image.

Coast—and even to the Rocky Mountains.

"I did all kinds of gambling. Slots, blackjack.... I went to Vegas on my way to Colorado. Saw the Hoover Dam. I knew Colorado was one of the best states because the governor was one of the first in this country to hire Japanese people. They were making automatic plumbing and they hired Japanese, the Nisei, Sansei. Even in 1946, after the war, after the internment. There was prejudice and many Japanese were fear, there were no jobs. But Colorado governor hired them to work in plumbing because the Japanese are hard worker."

Take went to Colorado in the early '70s to seek a potential business deal. "I had a friend, Mr. Mura, he was a branch manager at Yoshinoya. You know, they make the famous 'beef bowl.'" The popular network of restaurants features traditional Japanese cuisine in a fast-food environment. Take's friend showed him three stores in Colorado, encouraging him to join in. "I was thinking maybe to start a business there, but I was scared," Take admits. "It was too far away. Beef is so near there, close by, cheap. But there were rumors that business was bad. It was a dangerous trip and my first time in an airplane. We had to transfer, fly from Oakland to Burbank to Vegas, then to Denver. I was so scared, so scary! I kept imagined the accident. I was trying to sleep. My wife, she not afraid. But I was scared, every wind kept shaking and I was afraid." Take shakes his hands and laughs.

At the root of most of Take's business and moneymaking attempts and of many of Take's stories are the themes of fishing and food. But his tales are more unique than the typical fish story. "Have you ever seen a giant clam?" he asks. "We went to Bodega Bay, me and my friend and my wife and my friend's family. Dig in the mud for lots of clams. My friend's son started playing with the clams and the clam got angry and bit him!" We both laugh together at the comical image.

In another business scheme, Take and a bunch of friends decided to pool their money and build an eel pond where they would buy and feed and raise eels to sell to restaurants. The pond failed, he explains, because "everybody had no money!"

Launching into yet another of his moneymaking schemes, he goes on, "What about geoduck, have you seen geoduck?" Take asks for my notebook and scribbles a picture of the long, grotesque creature that I've eaten in Chinese restaurants—a huge white shellfish with a long neck that grows up to eight inches wide. "It's used in sushi at Japanese restaurants," he says, "but it has to be very fresh."

He explains, "I was in the geoduck exporting business. Well, sounds like big business, but really it was small business." During a fish worker's strike in Japan, Take and a friend hatched what appears to be truly a creative-but-harebrained idea: they would create their own import/export business and bring American geoduck to the seafood-deprived, strike-ridden Japanese. "There was a fish strike. They were only bringing bad fish, bad quality. Leaving it out all day." Take drove to Seattle to buy some geoduck and put it on a boat to Japan. "But the fish never made it to Japan. Someone must have ate it. So that was the end of the export business."

Once, Take says, he caught a fish and tried to send it airmail to his friend Nidochi in Japan. "You can't send a fish airmail!," I say.

Fishing was not only a business opportunity and a favorite pastime for Take and his wife, but also a way for him to bond with friends. His stories are littered with fishing references—for sardines up the California coast to Oregon, salmon in Seattle and trout in Lake David, near Reno. He reminisced about one lake trip where his friend cooked their catch over an open fire. "It was me, John and Thai guy. We knew each other from my restaurant and we were good friends. My Thai friend was very smart. We were friends for a long time. We fight so many times, but we still friends. We argued during the Vietnam War. He even called President Nixon once. He got a green card. He moved back to Thailand, and I don't know what happened to him."

Once, Take says, he caught a fish and tried to send it airmail to his friend Nidochi in Japan. "You can't send a fish airmail!" I say, and Take laughs. He starts to tell me about Nidochi, his best friend during his high school years. "He also did judo. We were sportsmen." Take's eyes light up when he talks about his friend, saying "so many stories..." Now, he says, his friend lives in a town in the mountains with hot springs.

Fishing eventually led Take to his most successful business venture—his own restaurant. He identified as a restaurant owner and a sushi chef. After his landscaping and gardening years, Take began working in Japanese restaurants as a dishwasher, the lowest position on the restaurant job hierarchy. By the '80s, Take had worked his way up and saved enough money to purchase his own restaurant, which he owned, managed and served in as a chef. The restaurant, Saffron, was located on 1666 Lombard Street in San Francisco's Marina District, only a few blocks from the bay.

"It was a rich neighborhood. I started with zero when I first came here. I always wanted to be a restaurant owner."

"Why?" I ask.

"It was a dream of mine from childhood," Take says. "My uncle owned a fish market, and I'd fish a lot. The fish wasn't fresh, though. It was in the countryside."

Saffron was a small restaurant. Take had three or four regular employees, new immigrants from Japan, doing many of the same jobs he had done when he worked in Japanese restaurants upon arriving in the U.S. Becoming a chef and restaurant owner was truly trial by fire for Take. "It was all the beginning," he says, things that he had never done before. "Even making sushi, I was learning." There was a liquor store owner on the block who soon became a close friend and a regular at Saffron, but the first time he ate there, Take has just opened up his new restaurant. He became so nervous about serving his new customer that he dropped some of the avocado for California rolls on the floor. "The guy saw it! I had to give him the sushi for free."

Soon Take was a seasoned restaurateur, waking up early each morning to hit the fish markets in San Francisco's Chinatown to check out their catch of the day. He draws me pictures of the knife and filleting methods he used to make bonito sashimi.

"Did your wife work with you at the restaurant?"

"Yes, she worked with me. We lived above the restaurant on Lombard Street."

"You must have been rich," I joked. "To own so much property!"

"No, no, not rich, not rich... We were poor. Business not too good. When I first arrived in America, I bought a home on Briggs Avenue in Alameda. I had good credit. Then I bought the building on Lombard Street and rented the house in Alameda. After I sold the restaurant, we moved back to Alameda. I sold the restaurant for $600,000. Made a profit. But I should have not bought the property on Lombard. There was property on Union Street that had a better value."

Despite Saffron's sixteen years of longevity, Take doesn't consider himself a success. "I didn't make enough," he says.

Take and I form a fast bond over our love of food. Our conversations about sushi and seafood quickly make me hungry—or even hungrier than

I already am. We meet after work, before I have a chance to eat dinner. The idea of food as more than sustenance—food as sharing, friendship—might partly be cultural, but through our common food interests I also get a sense of Take as he was in his restaurant business. He is exceedingly polite to me when we first meet, asking me if I would like a cup of coffee even though there isn't any coffee available in Clarendon Hall. Another evening after talking about our favorite dishes, he sighs and exclaims, "I wish I had a restaurant so I could serve you. I was the chef."

A lover of fresh fish, Take yearns for the food he can't have due to his dietary restrictions and the institutional menu at Laguna Honda. His weekly meals out with his wife are the one break he looks forward to. "The food here is so bad!" he says. "There's no flavor. Bland! Just spaghetti, no sandwiches, no Japanese food. Americans don't have flavor in their food." I agree and ask him what kinds of food he likes best.

"Chinese food."

"Really? Not Japanese food? Which dishes are your favorites?"

"The cheap ones," Take jokes. "Also I like chicken dishes. Sushi isn't bad for you but I didn't eat sushi. I ate pork! I think I ate too much yakitori. One time I was twenty-two, and a student friend took me to eat skewers of pork. More than twenty pieces!" It was his love of food that, in part, has affected his health. "That's why I had heart problems. There were no heart problems in my family. Just me. I ate too much. Not only yakitori, but also sausages. That's why I had too much trouble. My blood is no good. My kidneys, too."

In 2001, Take had a stroke. He was sixty years old.

Before his stroke, Take was in

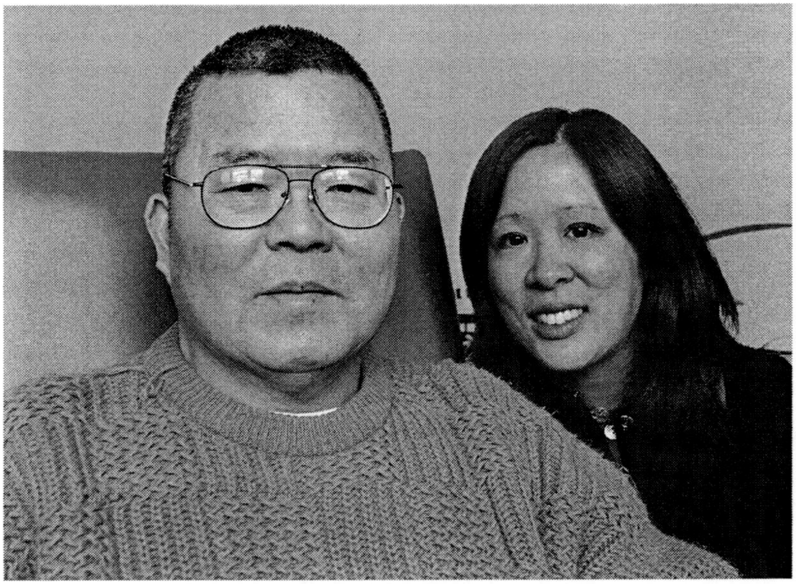

Takeshiro with his writer, Lisa

"Inside Laguna Honda is good, but outside no good. I want to be free."

decent health, although he had high cholesterol. "Sometimes I felt like my heart is something wrong," he says. "But symptoms never show up. I was not sure I was getting sick by heart attack. But I'm sure something wrong. I had a customer, a doctor. He save my life. Helped me discover something is wrong. The surgery, it had a eighty-five-percent success rate, a fifteen-percent failure rate. Very scary. He said, 'You shouldn't be existing in this world.' He told me when he touched my heart, my heart had problems already."

"So I had a triple bypass. After surgery you should be fine, but I am disability. My wife decided I was a disabled person and put me here at Laguna Honda. My brain was cut open four times. What was it? I don't know." Take says the brain surgery hasn't affected his memory too much, but a lot of his language skills have been lost, especially his English and writing skills.

Take moved to America for adventure. He planned on staying for a few years, maybe long enough to find a job and a wife. But he never planned on staying here for the rest of his life. "I didn't want to be here for so long," he says. "But it's too late, it's too late."

"Why is it too late?" I ask.

But we both know the answer. "I am old."

And he's here—in the hospital. Take talks about his sickness matter-of-factly, but says, "I don't want to be here."

He doesn't want to be in America, either. Or rather he wishes he were back in Japan. It's not that Take is anti-American. It's that he misses his native country. He misses it even more because he will most likely never go back.

The week before the 2004 presidential election, I mention that I might be late for our meeting next week because I need to go vote. "Are you going to vote?" I ask.

"No, I am not citizen. I have no plans to be one. I am permanent resident." He looks around him. "Inside Laguna Honda is good, but outside no good. I want to be free. I want to go wherever I want to. I want to leave here and go back to Japan."

"What do you think you would like to do if you were back in Japan?"

"I want to open a pharmacy and help other people with diabetes. Like I have. Diabetes people should eat a special diet food good for diabetes. I sell medicine for diabetes."

"That sounds like a good plan."

"That is my dream. I want to go back to Japan." Take suddenly looks up, excited about a new idea. "If you have extra money maybe you would invest in sending me back."

"Well, I don't have much extra money," I tell him. "But I wish I did."

Two weeks later, with our interviews now completed, I arrive to find two strange men in his room that I have never seen before. After some confusion, the nurses tell me that Take has moved into a new room down the hall. Unlike his old cramped two-room double, his new space is a large, airy single at the end of the hallway, away from the noise. There is a big window with a view of the Laguna Honda lawn, a precious commodity here. There is even room for all of his art supplies. Take is wearing a Christmas-themed green sweater, and is in good spirits, ready to have his picture taken for this volume. We wish each other happy holidays, but I feel sad, already imagining that he will miss my regular visits.

"Under the Golden Gate Bridge, when the baby whale was there with the mother and father? The situation was tearful. Please be sure to say that—tearful."

A few weeks later, I get a phone call from Take. "It's very important," he says. "I have some changes to my story. Under the Golden Gate Bridge, when the baby whale was there with the mother and father? The situation was tearful. Please be sure to say that—*tearful*."

"Of course," I say.

"Also, it was very dangerous area. Under the Golden Gate Bridge. Got to be careful."

I write this all down in my notebook. "I will be sure to mention that."

"Also, after I catch the whales, we fill the dead body with air. Drag it twenty miles away. The current is rough."

"Okay."

I ask Take if he has any advice for the people who will be reading his life story.

He thinks for a moment. "Don't eat whale meat," he says. "Because it is a very sad story. Very, very sad. Human society is fast to judge. But until husband die, disappear... very, very sad. Unlike pig and chicken and cow, they die in short time. But whales suffer more."

Who was Take, once upon a time? I have a great aunt who has been living in a coma in a hospital for nearly ten years. My mother and I visited her once. Her immediate family refuses to take her off life support, and she remains in a vegetative state, bloated by an IV drip, her growing hair clipped weekly by kind attendants. Nothing remains, at least visibly, of the woman who used to hand-knit baby sweaters for all her nieces and nephews, who survived a battle with breast cancer, who moved from China to Canada in middle age, raising two children on her own.

When I first meet Take I am overwhelmed with sympathy for him, this young "senior" stuck in a hospital in a country he never planned on growing old in, living apart from his wife whom he had planned on growing old with.

But Take is not like this. He is not silent, not confined. He is cranky and excited and angry and bitter and joyous like anyone else. He struggles to tell stories about his past, stories spanning oceans, rivers and lakes as well as his hopes for the future. "I am not like this!" he seems to be telling me. "I am more than this." In the end, I realize that which stories a person chooses to tell about him or herself, the way one chooses to define him or herself, is just as important as the stories themselves. What one chooses to include, or not include, and how one tells the story can be as revealing as its content.

When I first meet Take I am overwhelmed with sympathy for him, this young "senior" stuck in a hospital in a country he never planned on growing old in, living apart from his wife whom he had planned on growing old with. He is lonely, sad. He has no family except for his wife, no friends left to visit him here. When I am five minutes late for our meeting one week, he tells me, "I thought you had forgotten."

Yet it soon becomes apparent that Take has made his share of friends at Laguna Honda. As we walk down the hallways of Clarendon Hall, he says a friendly hello to everyone we pass—the tall man with a massive facial wound and bloody gauze, a petite woman balancing gingerly on her metal walker, the nurses that he knows by name. One night, when we are chatting in the library, Take suddenly stops talking and stands up from his chair, waving his arms at someone. I look up. His former art teacher is walking past us in the hallway. Take shouts out her name and they greet each other with hugs and smiles. Despite everything, he has found a home here.

When we walk past the nurses' station on his hall one evening, one of the nurses asks Take, "Did you meet your friend downstairs like you were going to?"

"Yes," Take says, motioning to me. "Lisa is my friend." ■

WRITER'S PROFILE

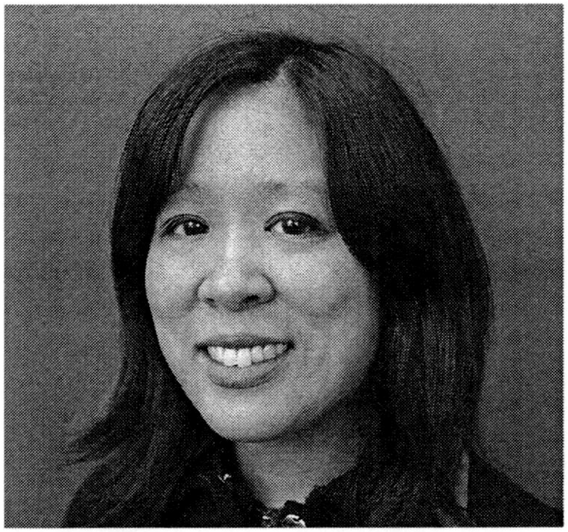

Lisa Ko

Writing has always been an act of preservation for me, a tool to counter amnesia. The only child of my parents and the only grandchild of my grandparents, I grew up as—and still am—the family observer, knowing that I was the only one who could remember our stories for the future.

As an adult, I have parlayed this knowledge into a career as a fiction writer, web writer for documentary films, and magazine editor, helping to tell stories on computer screens, television screens, and the printed page. I am also finishing up a master's degree in library science and archival studies, learning how to archive historic papers, letters, and photographs in order to save them from extinction, from being forgotten.

I am fascinated most of all by life stories: the anecdotes, the causes and effects, the ups and downs; the choices people make, the planned and more often than not, the unexpected. I always loved to hear the life histories of the elders in my own family, and was looking for a way to record and preserve others' stories when I first heard about the Life Stories Program.

Talking with Takeshiro Sakai was one of the most difficult and rewarding interviews I have ever done. I was overwhelmed by the emotional realities of his situation, frustrated by the language barrier, deeply affected by the parallels—and differences—between Take's life and that of my own family. Yet after each of our weekly meetings, I always felt that at the very least, I was being a friend to him, someone who listened in this crazy world. I hope that I have made a difference in his life as much as he has in mine.

Recommended Readings

If you'd like more information on how to get started in doing this type of life story work, here is a short annotated bibliography of selected works that might inspire and guide you. If you have other recommendations, please let us know at info@eldergivers.org.

Aging, spirituality, and working with elders:

From Age-ing to Sage-ing: A Profound New Vision of Growing Older by Zalman Schachter-Shalomi and Ronald S. Miller (Warner Books, 1995). The classic work in "spiritual eldering."

Vital Connections in Long-term Care: Spiritual Resources for Staff and Residents by Julie Barton, Marita Grudzen, and Ron Zielske. (Health Professions Press, 2003). Geared toward training people who work with nursing home residents, contains chapters on spiritual legacy (passing on the spirit of life), coming to terms with death and dying and recovering the self through the arts.

What Dying People Want: Practical Wisdom for the End of Life by David Kuhl, M.D. (Public Affairs, 2002). A well-known palliative care physician presents ways of finding new life in the process of dying, including a chapter on life review.

What's Worth Knowing by Wendy Lustbader. (Jeremy P. Tarcher/Putnam, 2001. These short vignettes with accompanying photos of older people, as told to geriatric social worker Wendy Lustbader, provide a legacy of wisdom on such topics as living well, time, later life, illness and frailty.

Fiction related to aging, elders and memory to inspire your creativity:

The Confessions of Max Tivoli by Andrew Sean Greer. (Farrar, Straus and Giroux, 2004). Another untraditional "love story" by a new San Francisco writer, which narrates the story of Max Tivoli, who grows older on the inside while the physical appearance of his body gets younger.

Lunch at the Piccadilly by Clyde Edgerton (Ballantine, 2003). A bittersweet fictional portrait of the characters in a North Carolina nursing home, described by Southern Living as "a zany tale about old folks and those who love them."

The Time Traveler's Wife by Audrey Niffenegger (Harvest Books/Harcourt, 2003). A captivating untraditional love story of a librarian who involuntarily travels through time, it has some profound questions about time and memory tucked in between beautiful writing and a very imaginative "structure."

Memoirs/non-fiction of elders and friendships with elders:

Am I Old Yet?: A True Story of a Timeless Friendship by Leah Komaiko (St. Martin's Griffin, 1999). A humorous and illuminating account of the friendship of the writer with a blind elder at the "California Chateau."

If I Live to Be 100: Lessons from the Centenarians by Neenah Ellis (Crown Publishers, 2002). Journalist Neenah Ellis recounts the lives of centenarians that she interviewed for an NPR radio program. She also describes the effects of interviewing elders, in this case, centenarians, on her own life and perceptions.

The Measure of My Days by Florida Scott-Maxwell (Penguin, 1968). An 80-year-old playwright and Jungian analyst assesses the predicament of old age.

No More Words: A Journal of My Mother, Anne Morrow Lindbergh by Reeve Lindbergh (2001, Simon & Schuster). The daughter of author Anne Morrow Lindbergh describes her experience caring for her mother, who was left nearly speechless by a stroke in her later years.

Old Friends by Tracy Kidder Houghton Mifflin, 1993). A beautiful journalistic and ethnographic portrayal of the life of two "old men" roommates in Linda Manor, a nursing home.

Tuesdays with Morrie: An Old Man, A Young Man, and Life's Greatest Lesson by Mitch Albom (Broadway Books, 2002). A dying professor shares his wisdom with a former student.

Oral histories and guides to doing them:

From Our Side of the Fence: Growing Up in America's Concentration Camps, edited by Brian Komei Dempster (Kearny Street Workshop, 2001). A wonderful collection of the experiences, in story and poem, of eleven Japanese-American elders who grew up in the internment camps.

Generations: A Century of Women Speak about Their Lives by Myriam Miedzian and Alisa Malinovich (Atlantic Monthly Press, 1997). This volume is organized in such a way as to highlight the differences in women's lives across generations—from first through third generation.

Legacy: A Step-by-Step Guide to Writing Personal History by Linda Spence. (Swallow Press, 1997). It's just what its title says, with some wonderful ideas for stimulating questions for elders.

Nine Lives: Uncovering the Wealth of Life Stories Within Our Nursing Homes – Volume 1, edited by Sarah J. Merrill (Eldergivers, 2003). This first volume of the Nine Lives Series contains the stories of nine elders, including a pioneering female surgeon and a blues musician.

Voices of Our Own: Mothers, Daughters, and Elders of the Tenderloin Tell Their Stories by Nancy Deutsch (San Francisco, 2001). Includes short oral histories and poems of San Francisco's Tenderloin residents, along with journal entries by the author/editor. A curriculum guide for intergenerational programs is also available.

Will the Circle Be Unbroken?: Reflections on Death, Rebirth, And Hunger for a Faith (New Press, New York, 2001); *American Dreams: Lost and Found* (New Press, 1999) by Studs Terkel. These are just a few of the classic works of America's "dean" of oral history, Studs Terkel.

About ELDERGIVERS

ELDERGIVERS is a San Francisco Bay Area organization celebrating 20 years of fostering positive connections between elders and the wider community. We accomplish this mission by identify, encouraging and cultivating the gifts of age and creating programs that allow the public easier access to the social, emotional, intellectual and spiritual resources of older adults.

North America's older generations have lived through incredibly tumultuous times and, as a result, have experience and perspective that can be drawn on to guide younger generations. Younger generations have, in turn, been immersed in an era of unprecedented technological change – change that has affected the breadth and depth of our knowledge and even the ways in which we relate to one another. Young and old need each other. The wisdom of age and the energy and spirit of adventure that characterize youth make a powerful combination.

ELDERGIVERS celebrates this reciprocity of gifts between the generations.

Our Volunteer Visitor Program links individuals from the community with elders who reside in nursing homes and other long-term care facilities. The faith-based version invites congregations to adopt nearby skilled nursing facilities and to provide one-to-one as well as group visits with residents. The program's secular counterpart makes vital connections between these residents and volunteers from corporations, public and private schools and affinity groups such as the Girl Scouts.

The A+ Program teams public and private schools (2nd through 12th grades) with senior residential sites and then pairs young and old in the context of a curriculum that helps the partners explore the subject of friendship.

Art With Elders places professional artists in nursing homes to teach residents how to paint and exhibits the product of these classes in an Annual Exhibit which is introduced to the public at a major arts venue in the Bay

Area. Following the inaugural event, the Annual Exhibit then travels to a variety of sites where it is enjoyed by more than 100,000 viewers annually.

Elder Arts Celebrations exhibits the visual arts of alumni, faculty and students over the age of 65 from Bay Area art schools and offers participants forums in which they can improve their abilities to present, exhibit and market their artwork and develop camaraderie among fellow artists.

Life Stories, the recent literary addition to ELDERGIVERS' art programs, attempts in a modest way to harvest the life-lessons of some of our society's most isolated seniors. Professional writers are introduced to selected nursing home residents for the purpose of capturing highlights of the elders' experience. These narratives are then edited and included in the *Nine Lives* book series.

ELDERGIVERS' programs are created and maintained to encourage on-going connections between the generations. They are based on "a reciprocity of gifts" – on the belief that every individual is of value and has something of value to share with others, no matter what their age or circumstance. If you are interested in being part of this adventure, we would welcome your inquiry and participation. Please contact us in any of the following ways:

Website	www.eldergivers.org
E-Mail	info@eldergivers.org
Voice Mail	415.441.2650 or 415.441.2649
Post	1755 Clay Street, San Francisco, CA 94109